Have the Birth You Want

Have the Birth You Want

Gill Thorn

HELP YOURSELF

British Library Cataloguing in Publication Data
A record for this book is available from the British Library

ISBN 0 340 78612 4

Typeset by Avon Dataset Ltd, Bidford-on-Avon, Warks

Printed and bound in Great Britain by
Bookmarque Ltd, Croydon, Surrey

Hodder & Stoughton
A Division of Hodder Headline Ltd
338 Euston Road
London NW1 3BH

Dedicated to my grandmother, Edith Harriet Lodge
1882–1970

In loving memory

Contents

Quick Guides

Acknowledgments

I am grateful to all the women who shared their birth stories with me and their strong sense that giving birth is something that women do for themselves, albeit with help. Special thanks to Clare Burt, whose personal journey provided the impetus for this book.

My thanks are also due to Mandy Hawke, who has supported women in their birth choices over many years; and to my daughters, Dr Joanna Thorn, a staunch advocate of women's rights, and Dr Annabel Corbett, a research psychologist who at the time of writing is expecting her first baby. They read the manuscript in its draft form and their patient, helpful and perceptive comments have been invaluable.

Introduction

It is strange how a single event can change the course of a life. My grandmother's experience of giving birth was so traumatic that she never had another child. She was eighty-seven, and I was expecting my first baby, when she told me what giving birth had been like for her.

My mother was born in 1911 – at home, as most babies were in those days. It was a long labour and as my grandmother recalled her experience I saw with astonishment that tears were running down her gentle face, soaking into her white linen handkerchief. It was the first and only time I saw her weep.

'The midwife made me have chloroform,' she said sadly. 'She pushed the mask on to my face. I didn't want it, but she forced me to have it.'

It was not the pain or the length of her labour that she found so unbearable, sixty years on. It was the memory of having control taken away from her, of being powerless to refuse sedation that she did not want.

My grandmother became a voluntary nursing sister during the First World War. She was strong, mentally and physically, invariably dignified and capable, but she could not bear the thought of having another child.

When it comes to labour, we are not really talking about science or even sense. We are talking about *feelings*.

Everyone agrees that women and babies should receive the best possible care during birth, but there are differences of opinion over what good care is and how it is best achieved. Women's views are often regarded as irrational, or of less importance than the views of health-care professionals, and women are sometimes put under a lot of pressure to follow other people's beliefs about what is best.

Nobody knows how defining a moment birth is until it happens. If a woman feels disempowered during this momentous experience it makes her doubt herself and her sense of loss can turn what should be joyous memories of the birth of her baby into a lasting torment.

How should a baby be born? As soon as one piece of research strikes a blow for natural birth another pushes mothers into the arms of doctors. Many women feel caught between the medicalised approach in vogue today and the ideal of natural childbirth; but there is no 'right' way to have a baby. Births are like dresses, different styles suit different women.

Some people place the highest priority on safety, regardless of the cost in human or economic terms; others feel that giving birth is exceptionally safe today and that choice is more important than further reducing the perinatal mortality rate by a fraction of a percentage point. Some women seek a totally pain-free labour; others are prepared to accept pain so long as it does not become overwhelming.

Having the birth you want matters because it contributes to physical and emotional wellbeing for you, your family and society in general. Quite simply, a good experience facilitates family bonding; a bad one hampers it. Patterns set up around the birth may be more lasting than previously thought.

For many women a satisfying birth, whether straightforward or complicated, easy or difficult, means retaining a sense of personal control. Losing the power to control your own life is something that cannot be put aside easily; and the resentment it leaves behind can be hard to get over.

If other people make decisions on your behalf you have to accept the consequences even if they are not what you expect. This is fine if you want this to happen, but if you are forced to give birth in a way that seems wrong to you, if other people take over with what they consider to be in your best interests, you may feel angry and cheated or, like my grandmother sixty years later, unbearably sad.

It has been suggested that women can feel a failure if they do not get the birth they want. I think that this underestimates them. An athlete who trains for four years to compete for an Olympic gold medal has no certainty of winning. No matter what you attempt, failure is a possibility, but you also acquire determination and self-belief. You learn more about yourself and you live more fully.

The reality of natural birth does not always to live up to the ideal. Drugs and technology have side effects and do not always make labour easier. An elective Caesarean section could be the best thing since disposable nappies, or leave you with an infection you could do without. A water birth at home may be a wonderful experience, or end in a transfer to hospital.

There are no guarantees that your plans will work out even when you have thought about birth and decided what is right for you; nor is it always somebody's fault when a birth turns out differently. When you share the decisions, however, you are not left with the fallout from a plan you never wanted.

Birthing women are not little girls asking the grown-ups to take away the bad things and make all the decisions for them. Those who choose to share decisions instead of putting themselves in the hands of others are capable of taking responsibility for this choice.

There is often a gap between what women hope for as regards birth and what they actually get. Bridging this gap takes knowledge and assertiveness. What you get depends on your decisions and preparations beforehand as well as your individual labour. If you are realistic and well-informed you are in a better position to make confident decisions and follow them through to achieve the birth you want, be it to avoid unnecessary intervention or to opt for an elective Caesarean section. Even when everything is not straightforward women overcome difficulties and achieve the birth they want.

Pregnancy is a time for gathering your strength, assembling the information you need and finding the people who can help you. It can take as much thought as the planning of any special event, but it can be equally rewarding.

A good birth experience usually involves a mother who feels empowered. It requires courage to face your own and other people's fears, to challenge inaccurate information, overcome opposition or make compromises. This book will help you to find out your options, plan your birth and then set out to achieve it.

1

A brief history of birth

Throughout history, rituals have been devised to manage uncertainty and ensure the health of the next generation. Society has always tried to control the wildness of women giving birth.

In the Middle Ages birth had no special status. Pregnancy was just a part of life, a normal experience for women. Remedies for cramp or sickness circulated like Chinese whispers and the expertise of a wise woman was sought to deal with problems. Birth could be lengthy, painful or even tragic, but incantations and spells, amulets and herbal remedies provided comfort and protection against the evil spirits that might harm a woman in labour or a newborn child.

As the influence of the Church grew, spells, amulets and herbal potions were outlawed as the trappings of witchcraft. The prayers and pilgrimages of religious devotion became the rocks to which women were encouraged to cling.

Today, the Church has lost much of its influence. Women still seek advice, but, instead of consulting a wise woman or a religious leader, they buy a book or a baby magazine and place their faith in a health professional with formal qualifications.

Risk management is central to the current way of thinking and in the developed world childbirth is no longer seen as a normal life event. Labour has taken on a potential for crisis and women readily submit to more and more intervention to avoid smaller and smaller risks. It is tempting to giggle or gasp at past rituals embraced by or imposed upon women in labour, yet some of today's medical routines will seem equally bizarre to future generations.

Constant social change is one of the lessons of history. Renewed interest in home birth, water for pain relief and the use of complementary therapies, alongside a consumer-led demand for Caesarean section, suggests we may be moving into a phase of greater diversity.

Hearth, home and hospital

During the Middle Ages, babies were usually born in the communal room of the house, where the mother could be kept warm. In rural parts of France, right up to the nineteenth century, it was common to give birth in the stable so that there would be no mess to clear up in the house. A stable provided warmth and privacy, soiled straw could be burned and other children would not be disturbed.

By the seventeenth century, women in more affluent households were able to retire to a bedroom within the house. Colonial American households partitioned a small room off the main room for use during labour. The 'borning room' contained a bed furnished with a straw mattress, often with a truckle bed slid underneath for a toddler or anyone caring for the mother to use.

The borning room was located behind the central chimney so that it was always warm, because warmth was considered essential during labour. Cold air, especially at night, might make the mother shiver and cause bleeding. The fire was stoked and the doors and windows stuffed with rags to prevent draughts. The heat would have been suffocating if labour lasted several days, but sealing the room prevented evil spirits from entering to harm the mother or the newborn child.

In many areas a labour was a social occasion. Everybody came to keep the mother's spirits up and enjoy a good gossip. Relatives and neighbours helped with tasks such as drawing and heating water, washing linen, preparing food, caring for small children and keeping the fire lively.

By the nineteenth century, some babies were born in hospital, but they were unsavoury places, only used by poor women who literally had nowhere else to go. These women were treated as medical guinea-pigs. Doctors went from dissecting room to ward and from bed to bed without washing their hands; as there was little understanding of the role of bacteria and no antibiotics, infection ran riot.

Thousands of poor women died of childbed fever; but many advances in the scientific and medical understanding of childbirth are founded on their sacrifice.

Attitudes to hospitals slowly changed in the twentieth century, when infection came under better control and powerful drugs for pain relief were introduced. First in America, then in Europe and Australia, giving birth at home came to be seen as old fashioned.

In 1965, about a third of all births in England and Wales took place at home. Five years later, the government produced the Peel Report, which was influential in encouraging the rise of a medical approach to childbirth. With no supporting evidence, it recommended that all births should take place in hospital. A building programme was undertaken to provide sufficient beds and by 1990 only one in a hundred births took place at home. Today, around 20 per cent of births take place at home in some areas of the UK. In other areas there are almost no home births.

Nearly all women used to give birth within or close to their home, where they felt safe. Today, many feel more secure giving birth in a hospital, with access to technology for monitoring labour and an epidural, a powerful method of pain relief that cannot be used at home. Technology requires higher staffing levels, however, and overworked midwives have no time to spend giving the reassurance and comfort that normally help a woman to cope with the challenge of birth.

Midwives and mothers

Midwifery is the art of being 'with women' and a good midwife does more than monitor a baby's welfare; she provides reassurance and support to give the mother strength and courage while she births her baby.

In the Middle Ages, communities usually chose a married woman for their midwife – preferably one with a large family, as she had greater personal experience of birth. It was considered improper for an unmarried girl to witness a birth.

The job description for the ideal midwife was simple: she must have attended a number of confinements without major mishap and be trusted to stay with the mother and help her as best she could. An early birth manual, *The Byrth of Mankynde*, published in 1545 advised:

> The midwife must instruct and comfort the party not only refreshing her with good meat and drink, but also with sweet words giving her hope of a speedy deliverance, encouraging . . . her to patience and tolerance . . .

The more births a midwife attended the more expert she became and her community came to rely on her. Some villages preferred their midwife to be post-menopausal for the practical reason that with no domestic ties she could be trusted to come quickly!

The stock-in-trade of the rural midwife included herbal remedies and amulets, supplemented with spells and incantations when labour proved difficult. Women felt comfortable with a woman of their own station in life who could be relied upon not to judge the household or ask for things they could not afford to provide. The midwife would enjoy the hospitality of the household and might receive a small gift such as a loaf of bread or a slice of ham, in gratitude.

Ideally, the midwife would take on an apprentice, a younger woman or sometimes her daughter, passing on both her skills and the job when she was too old or infirm to continue; but if she died prematurely women would help each other out until another mid-wife emerged whom they felt they could trust.

In the late sixteenth century, the witch hunts began. As Christianity spread and the influence of the priests grew, midwives were accused of witchcraft if a mother or baby came to harm, or even if they tried to relieve pain. In about 1591, Agnes Simpson used opium to relieve labour pain in England; in Scotland, Eufame MacCalzean cast a woman's pains on to a dog. Both were burnt at the stake.

Even more fanatical hunts took place in seventeenth-century Europe. One area of Germany is said to have put nine hundred witches to death in twelve months; and in Toulouse, France, four hundred were burnt at the stake in a single day.

The greatest zeal appears to have been reserved for midwives, often denounced by the doctors who were graduating from the new universities and struggling to gain power in the birth chamber.

If a labour was so difficult that the woman or child could not survive, a barber-surgeon was usually called. Barber-surgeons cost more than a midwife and they used surgical instruments, but gradually the more successful ones were asked to attend normal labours by those families who could afford them. The rise of the man-midwife in the seventeenth century helped to open the doors of the birth chamber to doctors.

Female midwives could be just as skilled, however. The first successful Caesarean section in the UK was performed by Mary Donally in 1738. She delivered a farmer's wife aged thirty-three, stitched her wound with silk, then dressed it with egg white. Mother and baby thrived.

The popular notion of a female midwife in the eighteenth to nineteenth centuries is of an untrained, uncaring, grimy charlatan frequently under the influence of drink. Some undoubtedly were, but many more were clean, kindly and able to provide comfort and simple herbal remedies. They knew if labour was progressing normally and sent for help when necessary.

At the beginning of the twentieth century, and as a direct result of war, midwives in Britain were regulated and obliged to undertake training. The government was so alarmed at the poor health of men conscripted to fight in the Boer War in 1899 that a health-care programme was introduced which included antenatal care. By 1902, an Act of Parliament made midwifery an independent profession with its own rules and regulations.

In America, however, the profession was all but extinguished as obstetricians came to dominate the labour ward and midwives were turned into obstetric nurses managing sophisticated technology and carrying out hospital regimes devised by doctors.

Today, American midwives are reclaiming their place as independent practitioners, the guardians of normal labour; but a problem faces the profession in many developed countries. When technology dominates the birth chamber midwives find it harder and harder to be 'with women' during birth.

Swinging from the chandelier?

Giving birth in the familiarity of her own home surrounded by people she knew well may have made it easier for a woman to listen to her own body and to choose the positions for labour and birth which she found most comfortable.

Prior to the eighteenth century, women rarely gave birth lying down: they might kneel, squat or stand, supported by other people; grasp a knotted rope or a sheet hung over the rafters; hang from their armpits, supported on the backs of two chairs; brace themselves on someone's lap; or even stand on their head with support for a short period.

Many women used a three- or four-legged birth stool, often carried from home to home by the midwife. Birth chairs give support without pressure during labour and the baby is born through the horseshoe-shaped hole in the seat. Their popularity has waxed and waned: fashionable in ancient times, they were reintroduced in Italy in the fifteenth century and used throughout Europe until about 1840, when they fell out of favour again.

When the benefits of upright positions for giving birth were rediscovered in the 1980s there was another flurry of interest and high-tech contraptions were developed, which resembled a dentist's chair into which a woman could be strapped and moved into various positions. These were not popular with women.

It became fashionable to deliver lying down on the bed during the late seventeenth century. This coincided with the rise of the man-midwife and may have been for his convenience, although women at that time often complained that they were bullied into kneeling or sitting by other women.

French women lay on their back in bed, propped up with pillows. Louis XVI is credited with getting women on to their backs to give birth by commanding his mistress to adopt this position so that he could see his child born in 1738. An illustration of a French delivery bed in 1743 shows two mattresses, the upper one doubled back and topped with a firm bolster at the head of the bed.

In England, women lay on their left side with a pillow between their knees and were delivered from behind. This was known throughout Europe as 'the English position'. Doctors considered it inconvenient, but women felt it saved their blushes and they could not see the instruments doctors used for a difficult delivery.

By the nineteenth century, women were encouraged to lie flat on their back, bracing their feet against a board placed at the foot of the bed or against the midwife's shoulders, or pulling on a piece of cloth looped round the foot of the bed. In hospital today many women still give birth lying on their back because nobody suggests any alternative. It is rarely an ideal position, but if technology or an epidural are used during labour they sometimes have no option.

Once the outlet to the birth canal (the perineum) came into view all sorts of things needed doing to it. Guarding it to prevent tears and cutting it to speed the delivery are manoeuvres made more necessary by the very position that brought the perineum into view in the first place!

Women having a natural labour today tend to use upright positions that enlist the help of gravity. They kneel, stand supported by helpers, semi-squat or sit as feels comfortable, changing position whenever they feel the need, like their forebears in the Middle Ages. The wheel has turned full circle.

A speedy delivery

An excessively long labour always has the potential to put the health of the mother and the baby at risk. Records from the sixteenth and seventeenth centuries show that some women delivered a healthy baby after labouring for two or more weeks, but every culture makes efforts to avoid this.

In the Middle Ages, the first line of defence was an amulet. Amulets are mentioned as far back as ancient Greece and were in common use in rural areas of Europe up to the nineteenth century. They could be of animal, mineral or vegetable origin; shaped like the uterus they were considered to have an affinity with it.

The rare and highly prized 'eagle' stone was about the size of a pigeon's egg and rattled like a nut in a nutshell, probably because a bit of mineral had come loose inside. It was found close to or actually in an eagle's nest, so its power was bound up with the symbolism of a mighty, free-flying, somewhat mysterious bird.

The next best substitute was a 'woman stone', a greenish pebble patterned with light and dark stripes. Like eagle stones, these were so precious they were often mounted in silver and treated as heirlooms. Less affluent women without access to such luxury objects put their faith in a hair ball from an animal's stomach.

The power of an amulet lay in its ability to draw the baby towards it. To prevent miscarriage it was hung around the neck. During labour, it was tied to the abdomen or the left thigh when pains were first felt, held on with a soft girdle or a lace and removed as soon as the baby was born. Correct placing was vital for it to be effective, and the ritual sounds remarkably similar to the positioning of a foetal heart monitor today. If the birth was prolonged no doubt the amulet was adjusted, just as today a midwife checks that a monitor is correctly placed.

Belief has a powerful psychological effect and feeling secure and protected helps a normal labour to progress smoothly, so an amulet tied on with a girdle would have inspired a woman in the Middle Ages as much as the electrodes of a foetal heart monitor held on with a webbing band reassures women today.

Before the witch hunts began, nobody enquired too closely if a midwife used an amulet or resorted to incantations or magic spells during a slow labour: they were too grateful for any help they could get. Amulets shared a bed with religion for decades and convents often kept a holy girdle, venerated as a relic, to attach them during birth. It reassured the faithful and could be lent to wealthy patrons.

In the seventeenth century, there was a resurgence of interest in herbal remedies, now regarded as medicines. Potions made from ergot, a substance obtained from mildewed rye, were given in broth or wine to strengthen contractions and speed labour up. Derivatives of ergot are used today to make the uterus contract.

Any substance that made the woman violently sick was also considered useful. Ipecacuanha, used by homoeopaths today as a remedy for pregnancy sickness, was valued for its ability to stimulate the uterus and speed up labour, but it was so costly that it was only available to wealthy women.

In the early eighteenth century, the new age of scientific discovery, medicines became cheaper and more widely available to women in the towns, before being brought by peddlers into the countryside. During the second half of the century, a profusion of new drugs were produced by chemical processes in the laboratory.

They were measured out into small glass phials with marks etched into the glass, so the dose was hit and miss, but they held out the promise of controlling the length of labour and eliminating pain. This goal was realised in the twentieth century with the development of technology to administer drugs and to monitor the baby's response with a degree of precision and safety unthinkable in the past.

So 'easy' has it become to hurry labour along, however, that it is sometimes encouraged on the flimsiest of pretexts; and with more regard for convenience than for the individual needs of a mother and baby.

Bearing the pain

Beliefs about the pain of childbirth have changed along with everything else. Medieval women believed it was caused by evil spirits, Christians saw it as a punishment for the sins of Eve. Today it is given a biological explanation.

Pain did not get much attention while the overriding concern was to ensure that both the mother and baby survived. It was simply regarded as inseparable from childbirth, an inevitable by-product of labour.

Christians saw any attempt to relieve pain in childbirth as contrary to the will of God. They cited 'Eve's Curse' – 'in sorrow thou shalt bring forth children' – and held out the promise that by suffering labour pain stoically a woman could attain the highly desirable 'state of grace'.

Given that pain relief prior to the nineteenth century could be hazardous, this may have been a helpful ideal, but by the mid-nineteenth century effective and relatively safe methods of dealing with pain had been developed for surgery. The Church, however, still condemned some women to struggle through long and difficult labours without respite.

Chloroform was first used during childbirth by Dr James Young Simpson, on the wife of one of his colleagues in 1847. She was so impressed by its effects that she named her daughter Anaesthesia. Six years later, it was administered to Queen Victoria in England during the birth of her eighth child, Prince Leopold. The drug could lead to loss of consciousness or even death and the dosage at the time was hardly accurate. Had any harm come to Victoria the history of pain relief for labour might have been set back by decades; but the Queen was enthusiastic and used it successfully again four years later at the birth of Princess Beatrice.

Celebrity endorsement can shift attitudes at a stroke! With Queen Victoria's endorsement, religious leaders reconsidered their opposition to pain relief for childbirth. By the turn of the century chloroform was in widespread use, while safer and more effective methods were being developed.

Even among Christians today, few women interpret labour pain as an atonement for the sins of Eve. Most people find the biological explanation more acceptable: that pain is a natural response when the muscle fibres of the uterus contract strongly and those of the cervix relax and stretch.

Some women regard pain during labour as unnecessary and avoidable, and do not see it as a moral issue. They are more than happy to take advantage of technology and drugs that make it a thing of the past. Others point out that drugs have unwanted side effects and technology increases the likelihood of further intervention (see Quick Guide, pages 71 and 72–73). They know that relaxation and complementary therapies help to release endorphins, the body's natural pain killers.

Does it matter what a woman puts her faith in if it helps her to feel secure and to handle the pain of her contractions?

Fathers and birth

For centuries birth was considered 'women's work' and in communities where there were women to be called upon men rarely entered the birth chamber. Women were considered to have more patience and experience; the father's presence was neither necessary nor seemly.

In isolated communities in America, Europe and Australia, however, where the lives of men and women were already closely entwined and mutually dependent, the father often stayed rather than leave his wife to give birth alone while he went to fetch female help. Even when a midwife arrived his strength might be needed to support his wife and if there was a problem he might be able to successfully apply knowledge gained from helping sheep to lamb or cows to calve. In 1588, colonist Jacob Nufer performed a Caesarean section on his wife, Elizabeth. She and her baby survived and she had another six children, all born normally.

Royal confinements were a different matter. The importance of succession meant that they usually took place in front of a jolly crowd of both sexes. Along with the women attendants, court advisors or members of the government would be present to witness that there was no skullduggery; a healthy newborn might be smuggled into the birth chamber, substituted for a child who died and illicitly proclaimed the royal heir.

Until the second half of the twentieth century, the majority of births took place at home. There was nothing to stop the father being present, but embarrassment and a sense of propriety persuaded most men that the 'decent thing' was to remain outside. The midwife might give him little tasks to keep him busy, such as boiling water or running errands, but in general men were considered to be, and believed themselves, surplus to requirements. In *The Care of Young Babies* published in 1940, Dr John Gibbens advised fathers: 'The right thing to do is to see your wife from time to time, to reassure her that all is well, that she is doing splendidly, and to leave the rest to your doctor. You can help him at this time by keeping anxious relatives away from the house.'

When a woman gave birth in hospital, her partner had no role at all to play. His job was to escort her to the hospital and make himself scarce. He was allowed to see her at visiting times, typically an hour in the afternoon (with other visitors) and an hour in the evening on his own. If he wanted to stay at other times he had to write to the consultant obstetrician and plead his case; unmarried partners, of course, need not even bother to apply. The doctor was the final arbiter of whether a father could be present when his child was born.

In the 1970s, new technology changed the role of the midwife. The Cardiff infusion pump, for example, was a complex and rather unreliable machine that measured the strength of a woman's contractions and automatically infused drugs to accelerate her labour. An alarm sounded if there was any problem so a midwife could supervise several women at the same time. Midwives flitted from bed to bed looking after machinery, but spending less time offering comfort and support.

For much of history fathers were banished from the birth room but, like the farmers of the last century, they were now needed.

Women found it distressing to be left alone for long periods during labour. Suddenly fathers had a role again.

Even men who had no wish to be present at a birth and no knowledge of what would happen or how to support their partner were pressed into service as companions and comforters. While some said they would not have missed the birth of their baby for the world and that it strengthened their family ties, others found the experience traumatic.

Fathers have always been expected to do 'the decent thing'. Currently this means being present and supportive during the birth, not leaving it all to the professionals. A father who tries to wriggle out of his supporting role is seen by some people as 'letting his partner down'; but, at the same time, there is a lively debate as to whether women are instinctively better at the role of birth partner.

The change in attitude to men's presence when women give birth is a good example of how social and cultural ideals shape birth as much as physical factors.

Doctors and birth

From the Middle Ages until relatively recently, most women preferred to be attended by midwives rather than doctors. When labour required tender loving care and a pair of hands to catch the baby, midwives were more than competent.

Doctors in the sixteenth century were called only in extreme circumstances. They were generally of a higher social class, their book learning and their instruments set them apart, and they had to be paid more. It was when a birth was really difficult or the life of a mother or baby was in peril that a doctor might save the day.

Unlike midwives, doctors did not want to sit around waiting for a baby to put in an appearance in its own good time when a slow delivery could be hastened with instruments. Using instruments gave them something to do, something active and more saleable than the herbal tea and sympathy served up by midwives.

The Church did not allow women to study medicine at the newly established universities and while women accused of witchcraft were being burnt at the stake en masse in Europe it was often the testimony of a doctor that sealed the fate of a midwife. At this time a power-battle was going on in England between midwives, doctors of the newly formed Royal College of Physicians and the barber-surgeons.

In about 1588, a barber-surgeon called Peter Chamberlen invented forceps, essentially a pair of oversized, hollow spoons. Spoons were already used frequently by both midwives and barber-surgeons to assist a difficult birth but, crucially, Chamberlen invented a device that locked them together so that they could not damage the baby's skull. It was this that revolutionised childbirth by saving babies who were presenting with unusual difficulties.

The invention proved extremely profitable. Peter and his brother attended the ladies of the English court and travelled around Europe charging huge fees for their services. Mindless of the benefits to women in general, they went to great lengths to keep their secret within the family, surrounding it with drama and mystery in a performance that must have terrified the poor mother. Two men brought in a large carved and gilded box. The brothers blindfolded the mother, banished all her female attendants including the midwife and disguised the sound of metal by ringing bells and drumming on the floor with sticks. The secret remained in the family until the latter part of the seventeenth century, when other doctors developed similar expertise.

In the early eighteenth century, however, barber-surgeons lost the right to attend women in labour. University-educated doctors with access to newly discovered medicines as well as surgical instruments took over. Their growing influence stemmed from their skill at resolving previously fatal complications, although they were not always very successful.

Caesarean section, for example, has been practised for over two thousand years. Women were expected to survive in early Egyptian and Jewish communities, but the skills then seem to have been lost until the Middle Ages. In extreme situations, women successfully performed Caesarean sections on themselves and up to 1888, according to the American medical historian R. P. Harris, 66 per cent survived their own surgery. Doctors could only achieve 33.5 per cent survival in America and 14 per cent in Britain.

The nineteenth century saw the rapid advance of a belief in science over religion. As understanding of physiology grew and new drugs were developed the influence of doctors over childbirth also grew, and in the twentieth century there was a new solution to the uncertainties of labour: control by technology.

A woman became a patient and her body became a doctor's field of practice. Childbirth was no longer seen as a normal life event.

The rise and rise of technology

Technology provides genuine solutions to certain problems, but it also makes money for the firms who develop, manufacture and maintain it and it empowers the doctors whose skills and patient-base are needed to use it. Whether we like it or not, profit and power are major forces that drive its use in labour.

Companies take out patents to protect their investment and their future profits just as the Chamberlen family deliberately kept the design of forceps a secret for over a hundred years. When a new drug or piece of technology becomes mainstream more profit is made, so there is in-built conflict between restricting something to essential use and the profit incentive which would like it to be used as widely as possible.

Profit provides the incentive to plug technology, but it is not just a case of toys for the boys. More is seen to be done by adding something than by taking it away, so everyone is seduced. Instruments gave eighteenth-century doctors something to promote and allowed them to charge higher fees. By the same token, high-tech labour is easier to 'sell' than natural birth where there is no value to be added.

When technology is used too widely, however, disturbing side effects are often revealed. Monitoring babies electronically, for example, has been found to increase the Caesarean section rate without benefiting mothers or babies. In many developed countries at least twice as many operations are performed as can be justified by better health or reductions in mortality.

Technology also affects what is seen as normal labour. The concept of time became important to daily life during the Industrial Revolution when clocks were used as a means of running the factories smoothly; but timing the length and frequency of contractions and the duration of labour begs the question: what is normal? A counting exercise was used to answer this.

In the 1950s an American, Emanuel Friedman, gathered data about the rate of dilatation achieved by women labouring in hospital, which he plotted on graphs. He found that the average woman's cervix dilated about one centimetre per hour so the average labour lasted around twelve hours. Confusing *statistical* normality (what he observed) with *physiological* normality (what ought to happen), he suggested that anything outside his statistical average was 'probably abnormal'. Friedman's curve became the standard way of measuring progress in labour.

Plotting progress on a chart promises more control, so 'partograms' were devised to show the average rate of dilatation and descent of the baby's head. As soon as these charts were interpreted as indicating 'normal' labour it was only a short leap to the notion that any labour deviating from the chart needed correction.

In the 1960s, labour was considered prolonged if it lasted more than thirty-six hours. By the mid 1970s, drugs and technology had been developed to speed up contractions and the definition of 'prolonged labour' shrank to twenty-four hours. Ten years later, 'normal birth' had been redefined and many midwives and women expected birth to take no longer than about twelve hours. Technology was available to accelerate any labour that seemed to be dawdling.

Speeding up labour can make contractions more painful, however, and some babies become distressed. More drugs and technology can be used to solve these problems and more profit is made; but it takes women further away from self-determination and creates more dependence on doctors.

While technological advances have certainly played a part in making childbirth safer they have also taken away women's confidence in their ability to give birth unaided. When normal labour is seen as a high-risk endeavour rather than an ordinary bodily function like breathing or running, the main beneficiary may be the medical technology industry.

Women's ways of knowing

New regimes tend to discredit old beliefs in order to strengthen their own influence, but in doing so they often get rid of the baby with the bath water. Today, parents and professionals feel reassured by science, just as past generations put their faith in witchcraft or religion. When any set of beliefs is widely accepted, however, it can be difficult for individuals to express a different opinion. Querying the 'truths' of science is no easier today than it was for a woman in the seventeenth and eighteenth centuries to question the authority of the priests.

Valuable though it is, science makes a poor job of taking feelings into account and it is not as objective as everyone likes to think. Health professionals sometimes rely on research evidence of dubious quality because it backs up their 'gut' feeling or personal preference. It also focuses on separate parts rather than the whole person: midwives log what happens hour by hour during labour, making decisions based on what they expect to happen next and what a machine shows.

Overrating science can devalue intuition, a more holistic sort of knowledge that suits the connected, co-operative ways of working that many women prefer. Measuring and recording may help a midwife to feel in control, but she cannot get to know a woman by ticking boxes. Intuition can provide insights that science cannot, but it does not flourish if care is fragmented, or if women are separated from their instincts by what the scan or the monitor says.

Like science, intuition is founded on observation, but seeing through a child's eye. A child sees 'all' rather than filtering data and making assumptions in the way an adult may. When you get to know someone well you judge how they are feeling from a whole range of clues: body language, the sound of their voice and what they leave out as well as what they say. In a strange way you know them all the time: even if you have not seen them for some time a sudden thought or a feeling relating to them may flash into your mind.

Physical or 'true' intuition provides knowledge that on examination proves to be right. It arrives suddenly without a rational thought process and is preceded or accompanied by a physical sign that you learn to interpret. It is not under conscious control and it is not the same as wanting something to be the case: the feeling is qualitatively different and you recognise it when it comes. If everything is in place true intuitions 'happen'; they do not have to be sought.

You may think you know something 'intuitively' if the logic is impeccable: for example, that it is safer to have a baby in hospital because all the equipment is to hand; but however obvious it may seem it does not stand up to scrutiny.

True intuition can be backed up by research evidence and good research is built on intuitive thought. Nobody expects science to give the right answer every time; nor is all science discredited because some of it is of poor quality or produces false truths. If we apply the same standards to knowledge provided by intuition it can be an equally valuable way to guide decision making.

Neither science nor intuition has a monopoly on truth: either can be right or wrong. Technology helps some women to give birth; a strong belief in the body's ability to give birth without harm, to do the job for which it is designed, helps others.

Marrying the clarity of science with the deep 'knowing' of intuition might help more women to have the birth they want; but this begs an age-old question: who should be in charge of childbirth?

Controlling nature, controlling women

Until relatively recently, the politics of the birth chamber have been waged between professionals over the heads of mothers, who were expected not to have opinions but to do as they were told. The ideal patient put her faith in her doctor and followed his advice to the letter. Treated like gods, some doctors grew into the role and rarely questioned the wisdom of their own advice.

Forty years ago when a woman entered hospital her pubic hair was shaved off 'to reduce infection'. She was handed a hospital gown to wear, given an enema 'to make space for the baby' and obliged to take a bath. With her clothes removed and her partner banished she became a dependent patient, not a woman capable of giving birth as nature intended.

She lay passively in bed waiting to be told what to do by a midwife or doctor who knew more about her labour than she did. She was denied food and given pain-relieving drugs so that she did not cry out and upset the rows of other women in her ward. Her baby was delivered for her while she lay on her back on the bed, because that was convenient for the professionals attending her.

Today, a woman giving birth in hospital wears her own clothes and has her own room with her partner in attendance. She can move about and eat if she wishes, but she may be strapped to a foetal heart monitor to give a base reading of her baby's heartbeat and be examined internally every four hours to check 'progress'.

Midwives feel more secure following known procedures, which are useful ways of keeping tabs on individual women when a ward is busy, but base readings and four-hourly internal examinations are not essential to giving birth. They do not happen when a baby is born at home. Like the stoked fires and amulets of earlier times, these routines ease uncertainty; and in a hundred years' time history may judge them as further efforts to control nature by controlling women.

Thirty years ago, the majority of first-time mothers had an episiotomy, a cut in the birth outlet. Nobody questioned that this was best for them, that it was easier to stitch and would prevent a tear or a prolapse later on, although there was no evidence for this assumption. There are several reasons why an episiotomy might be necessary, including the skill of the midwife and the position the woman adopts for delivery. It was discovered, however, that women had a considerably higher chance of 'needing' an episiotomy when the medical team was in favour of them. The 'need' depended largely on the views of the consultant!

In the late 1970s, women began to object to routine episiotomies and to being forced to give birth lying on their back. They wanted to use alternative positions such as kneeling or squatting; they wanted to be in charge, and saw no reason to comply with what they regarded as paternalistic control. In 1982, an obstetrician at the Royal Free Hospital in London refused to allow his patients to adopt any birth position other than lying on their back. Coach loads of women highlighted the issue by demonstrating vociferously in London.

Women doctors were also at risk of paternalistic control. In 1987, after a series of secret meetings to which she was not invited, colleagues of Dr Patte Coombes, an American GP, revoked her right to deliver babies in the local hospital.

What really upset her colleagues was her support for a woman's right to self-determination. If a woman refused an ultrasound scan or a mother with a breech baby did not want to see a consultant obstetrician as required by the protocol of the hospital, Patte Coombes accepted the decision. In so doing she threatened the power-base of her hospital-based colleagues. They claimed her work was 'in flagrant violation of good standards of care', although she had delivered four thousand babies without losing a mother or child. Challenged about her superb safety record they said she had simply been lucky!

In a similar case in Britain in 1986, obstetrician Wendy Savage broke ranks by supporting the rights of women and her fellow consultants responded by attacking her credibility. In each case the accusers were forced to back down by the overwhelming force of evidence.

A woman's choice

The practices surrounding birth change along with the beliefs of the whole of a society. Against a background of witchcraft and evil spirits women in the Middle Ages put their faith in amulets and some useless or harmful herbal potions; but they also used raspberry-leaf tea and concoctions of ginger which have stood the test of time and are still in use today.

The Church discredited these old remedies and women turned to devotion to saints. The emotional support of prayer and the promise of attaining a state of grace through forbearance undoubtedly helped them to handle a normal birth, but it was of less use when there was a genuine complication.

Science discredited spiritual comfort in favour of new treatments. Pregnancy became a relentless search for problems rather than a celebration of new life. Many women are still convinced that evidence-based medicine has all the answers and every problem can be fixed by a drug or a piece of technology.

Since the 1970s, however, there has been a huge increase in the amount of information available to women about childbirth. Choice in the past has often been defined by what the doctor or midwife felt to be the best course of action, but the place of women in society has shifted and they are more confident about asking for what they want. Birthing women are not as compliant as they used to be.

Medical advances, improvements in social welfare and better living standards have revolutionised birth in the developed world, but the more power the guardians of a belief system have the more is expected of them. Change tends to occur when disillusionment sets in.

Safety, although always important, is no longer an overriding issue for a healthy woman. Parents shopping for a pushchair expect to be shown several models that comply with safety regulations, not to be told what colour or style they should buy; and they want health professionals to ensure a safe birth, but not to dictate where or how their baby will be born. Women now see themselves as consumers, not patients. Where something is an option rather than essential they see no reason why it should not be their choice.

In brief

- The history of childbirth shows that social and cultural factors have as much influence on childbirth as physical factors. Each era improves some things at the expense of others.
- Childbirth rituals are entwined with the wider concerns of a society and priorities change; practices considered essential by one generation are cast aside by the next and replaced with new rituals.
- Science is highly valued at present so it can be hard to challenge, but it is not the only source of knowledge; intuition can be equally useful.
- History supports the notion that there is no one right way to give birth. There is plenty of room for diversity and individuality.

2

The natural process

The female body is fine-tuned for childbirth, but the only fixed element in labour is the basic physiology. Nature has shaped this over thousands of years by the cruel, but effective means of natural selection: the genes of women who were able to give birth successfully were passed on.

Natural birth is a triumph of engineering and chemistry backed up by instinct, and the whole process is sufficiently well-designed and versatile to work for most women, most of the time. Hormones and your choice of position enlarge the capacity of your pelvis. Your contractions coax your baby into the best position and shape her head to fit the birth passage. The skull bones overlap spontaneously and her body twists to negotiate what seems an impossibly small space.

Viewing labour as the efficient extraction of a baby from a mother ignores the human side of the experience, however. Labour is controlled by your brain via your hormone system, which in turn is affected by how you feel. If you are relaxed and confident your body can work to its maximum efficiency, but some women labour faster than others, just as some have the stamina to run long distance while others are better at sprinting. Giving birth can never be a purely mechanical process.

The more you understand about the birth process the more confident you will feel about your body's natural ability to deliver your baby safely. Normal labour is not always as swift or as easy as you might wish; but neither is it the nightmare that some women seem to expect. With good support, most women find they can meet the challenge.

Even though ways have been developed to speed up contractions, take away pain or bypass the birth process altogether for women who need or want this, the human race would never have survived if the majority of women were not able to give birth unaided. Regaining confidence in the female body is a challenge for parents and professionals alike.

Cradled in the pelvis

Your pelvis is part of the bony infrastructure that supports your body. It allows you to walk upright and provides attachment points for the muscles that control your limbs and torso. It has three main bones, the sacrum at the back and the two iliac (hip) bones which curve round your sides to meet at the sacroiliac joint. The top of this joint and the front of the iliac bones form your pubic bone, the front of the inlet to your pelvic cavity. Your pelvic floor supports your internal organs and the whole structure forms the perfect cradle for your baby.

To trace the shape of your pelvis, feel your hip bones on either side, then take your hands round your back and feel the curve of your sacrum. Follow it down between the cleft of your buttocks to feel your coccyx, the small bony tail of your spine. Take your hands down the front side of your hip bones to your pubic bone. The iliac bones separate here to form your pubic arch, which is shaped like a wishbone around your clitoris and vulva.

The space between your coccyx and your pubic arch is the outlet of your pelvic cavity through which your baby passes to be born. It may seem dauntingly small, but your body has various mechanisms to give your baby extra room. This adaptability enables most women to give birth successfully, no matter what their size or that of their baby.

The cavity of your pelvis is like a short, curved cylinder with the lower segment of your uterus fitting snugly into its brim. The inlet is wider from side to side while the outlet is wider from front to back.

Your baby's head is wider from front to back and her shoulders are wider from side to side, so she twists to negotiate your pelvis. When she lies with her back towards your front, the best position for birth, she enters your pelvis facing sideways to match the shape of the brim, turns to fit under your pubic arch and emerges facing your back. At the same time, her body enters the brim with her back to your pubic bone and turns sideways to pass through your pubic arch.

During pregnancy, hormones are secreted in increasing quantities to soften your ligaments, the tough, fibrous connective tissue that links bones. This allows more movement in the sacroiliac joints, which connect your pelvis to your sacrum, and in the symphysis pubis, which connects the iliac bones at the front. Your pubic arch can expand by more than a centimetre during labour.

Moving your body freely adds to the help given by hormones. If you stretch your thighs apart, for example, your sacroiliac joint widens naturally. When your upper spine moves in one direction your sacrum moves in the other, so if you lean back from the waist your tail tucks in, closing your pelvic cavity; but if you lean forward your sacrum swings back and your pelvis opens.

A baby's brain is like dense foam rubber protected by the firm but flexible skull bones. These bones are linked with 'seams' of tissue, like tough canvas, that can overlap during birth without harming the brain. Your contractions and the muscles of your pelvic floor mould your baby's head to fit through your pubic arch. In the weeks after birth the seams fuse, leaving the diamond-shaped fontanelles, or soft spots, which gradually disappear as your baby grows.

At home in the uterus

Supported by your pelvis, your baby is able to grow snugly enfolded in her first home. By the end of pregnancy, your uterus is about the size and weight of a large melon, with walls as thin as melon rind, yet muscular enough to hold on to your baby for nine months before opening for a few hours to push her out.

The uterus is made up of layers of involuntary or smooth muscle, the sort that enables your heart to contract and relax automatically. Smooth muscle is controlled by hormones so that it can carry out the body's essential housekeeping tasks with no effort on your part, leaving you free to concentrate on other things. Unlike skeletal muscle which is under voluntary control – you can decide to walk faster to arrive somewhere on time – you cannot speed up labour by an effort of will.

The individual muscle fibres of the uterus contract automatically throughout your life to maintain its tone and to keep it healthy; but each fibre acts independently and in order to deliver a baby they need to work together. A few weeks after conception hormones start to 'wire up' or co-ordinate the individual muscle fibres. As the process gathers momentum you may feel painless 'Braxton Hicks' or practice contractions, or notice that your uterus feels firm as a football for a few seconds.

Braxton Hicks contractions occur randomly at first but, like novice American line dancers, they gradually take on a rhythm as the muscle fibres start to work together. The contractions of early labour feel pretty similar, but as the wiring up nears completion and the uterus functions as one giant muscle they become co-ordinated and stronger.

Your baby passes into the birth canal through your cervix, which is formed mainly of horizontal fibres and stretchy connective tissue. Your cervix is like a tube, about three centimetres long and sealed with a mucus plug. One end or 'os' leads to the uterus and the other to the vagina. Before you go into labour, the hormones that kept it closed during pregnancy are withdrawn and replaced by prosta-glandins to soften or 'ripen' it.

In a first labour the inner os usually disappears or effaces before the outer os starts to dilate, just like stretching a new polo-neck jersey over your head. If you have already had a baby, your cervix may efface and dilate at the same time, more like pulling on a well-loved jersey. The membranes of the amniotic sac (bag of waters) detach partially from the uterus and the mucus plug or 'show' comes away.

During labour, the individual muscle fibres shorten with each contraction, so that the space inside your uterus gets smaller and your baby is pressed gently and persistently against your cervix to help to dilate it.

The upper segment of the uterus has a greater proportion of longitudinal muscle fibres which contract more strongly; so, while the upper segment thickens, the area around the cervix thins out and opens up.

Contractions do more than simply open your cervix and push your baby out, however. Smooth muscle is like latex: the more it is stretched the more strongly it contracts. If your baby's head is at an angle it stretches one area of the uterus more and produces stronger contractions in that area. This helps to tuck your baby's head in so that she is in a better position to pass through your pelvis.

The muscle layers of the uterus act rather like the structure of a trampoline, which is designed to help the trampolinist to land centrally, ready for the next jump. Anything firm placed under one area of a trampoline prevents this and similarly pressure from the belt of a foetal heart monitor, or the mother's spine if she lies on her back, can prevent the uterus from contracting effectively.

Your baby needs a good supply of oxygen until she is born and can take air into her lungs, so the muscle cells in the area of the placenta grow bigger, stretch less and do not contract as strongly. This area of the uterus receives more of the hormones that damp down contractions during pregnancy, possibly secreted by the baby. When she is born and her cord stops pulsating, or is tied and cut, the area contracts strongly in order to deliver the placenta.

Bathed in hormones

Hormones provide the delicate mechanism that begins by preparing your uterus for labour, keeps it working smoothly for as long as necessary and ends with the birth of your baby. They are closely related 'families' of chemical substances secreted by glands to regulate the way that other organs function. They control physiological responses and the rational behaviour that distinguishes humans from animals.

Hormones are responsible for the way that your uterus is able to hold on to the rapidly growing baby for the nine months of pregnancy, then reverse its action completely by letting the baby go after the relatively short period of labour.

Your brain is physically connected to other parts of your body by nerves that act like a telephone network, sending rapid responses by a series of impulses. The message that something is painful flashes back so fast it is virtually automatic and this gives you time to judge the entire situation and decide what to do. Your brain then sends instructions such as 'move your body' via your hormone system.

Some hormones pass messages as fast as nerves: for example, fear floods your body with adrenalin ready for fight or flight. Others are complex, act more slowly, compete for the same receptors and carry different messages. For example, oestrogen increases your sex drive when it taps into your brain's receptor cells, but it tells the uterus to prepare for an egg and it makes bones absorb calcium from your blood.

Hormones can be transmitted in different ways. The saliva glands use ducts to carry them for local use while the thyroid gland pours them directly into your bloodstream. Ovaries and testicles use both methods.

Glands control the day to day instructions which keep your body working effortlessly, and the instructions necessary to achieve something occasional but dramatic, such as giving birth. They never act independently but perform a delicate balancing act, regulating their output to the levels your brain judges to be 'right' for a particular situation.

The body's hormone system is also the interface between emotions and actions, providing the link between how you experience and interpret the world and your actions. By controlling and balancing the secretion of hormones your brain oversees your behaviour. Your personality and your past and present experiences determine what your brain judges to be the 'right' thing to do.

The part of your brain that provides the link between the two systems, matching your feelings and actions with how your brain interprets the world, is your hypothalamus. This is the commander, so to speak, that controls your pituitary gland which in turn controls the output of your endocrine glands.

If your body was a dress factory, your brain would be the chief executive predicting next season's fashions and deciding which to manufacture; your hypothalamus would be the manager in charge of getting the right fabrics and trimmings; your pituitary gland would be the supervisor overseeing the staff and your endocrine glands would be the machinists and finishers obeying orders.

When your brain decides you should be alert it secretes stress hormones, to help you adapt to and learn from a new situation. Too much stress can be bad but the right amount helps survival. The stress hormones ACTH, Beta-endorphin and cortisol (see box, page 34) help your baby to cope with delivery and respond to her new environment. The rise in the level of these hormones may signal your body to prepare for labour.

Hidden in your brain behind your eyes is an internal clock, set by darkness and daylight but affected to some extent by habit. It regulates your body rhythms, the twenty-four-hour routine of sleep, temperature, hormone output and so on. Output of hormones such as cortisol reduces from about 4 p.m., to conserve production at night when you are less likely to need to be alert, and steps up again in the early hours of the morning. By the time you awake your hormones are at their daytime levels again.

Circadian rhythms may influence the start of labour. Although doctors claim that births occur randomly throughout the day and night, many women say that labour started during the hours of darkness. Some feel contractions for several evenings in succession

Birth hormones

Oestrogen is made by your ovaries and the placenta. It helps your body to use calcium and prepares your uterus for labour by wiring the individual muscle fibres up so they work together. High levels of oestrogen are needed for normal labour.

Adrenocorticotropic hormone (ACTH) prepares your mind and your body for action. It makes you more alert and it triggers the production of cortisol.

Cortisol releases fats and amino acids from storage sites in the body to give you the raw material for dealing with stress. High levels switch your body's resources from growth and repair to short-term survival. The surge produced by labour releases extra lung surfactant, a substance that primes your baby to breathe air.

Beta-endorphin is one of a group of anti-stress hormones that give pleasure. It is released along with cortisol and it helps to regulate female sex hormones, such as oestrogen, by blocking instructions to your ovaries. It can delay labour to give you time to relax if you are under mild stress and it can take the edge off pain.

Oxytocin makes muscles contract during orgasm, labour and breastfeeding (when stored milk is 'let down' for the baby). It helps you to fall in love with your partner or your baby. Towards the end of pregnancy your baby releases oxytocin, which may also help to trigger labour.

before finally going into labour, perhaps because their naturally lower cortisol levels at this time help them release oestrogen.

Your brain tells your ovaries to produce more oestrogen to finish wiring up your uterus so that it can contract strongly. At the same time, your progesterone levels decrease, removing the hormonal brakes that stopped contractions during pregnancy, and prostaglandins soften up your cervix to make it stretch more easily.

When your brain judges everything to be 'right', your hypothalamus tells your pituitary gland to secrete oxytocin, your contractions strengthen and labour begins.

Born naturally

When you are ready to go into labour, your uterus is like a car prepared for a journey, with the engine running and the gears in neutral. Your hypothalamus is the driver and your hormones control your contractions in the same way that the brake and accelerator control the motion of a car.

Surprisingly, it is not known exactly what starts labour off, but the trigger may come from your baby rather than you. Ideally, several things need to be right before labour begins, including a baby who is mature enough to survive and surroundings where you feel secure and relaxed enough for labour to take place.

Progesterone damps down contractions and when this is withdrawn the brakes are released and oxytocin is secreted to act as the accelerator. Contractions are usually slow and gentle at first, but the rhythm of labour builds up like Ravel's *Bolero*, the music made famous by skaters Torville and Dean in the 1980s. Each contraction hugs your baby, but leaves her with slightly less space and so, to spare her having to cope with bear hugs for too long, the contractions become stronger and more frequent, dilating your cervix faster.

The more favourable your baby's position the quicker your cervix is likely to open. As it dilates, your pituitary gland secretes more and more oxytocin to keep the process going. Endorphins, released in increasing quantities to take the edge off pain, can make you feel spaced-out or reluctant to be disturbed in any way.

When your cervix has opened sufficiently, your baby passes from the uterus into the birth canal. Persistent pressure against the banana-shaped muscles of your pelvic floor aligns her head with your pubic arch. The pelvic floor muscles stretch apart to let your baby pass through and this stretching triggers pushing contractions.

Your body floods with adrenalin to provide a surge of energy and stimulate the final expulsive reflex that delivers your baby.

After a natural labour, the cocktail of birth hormones makes you and your baby alert, wide-eyed and especially responsive to each other. Eye contact, so important when falling in love, helps to forge the bond between you. Meanwhile, the placenta separates and the blood vessels seal to prevent haemorrhage. Over the next few days more contractions shrink your uterus to its pre-pregnant size.

Roller-coaster ride

Labour is not simply a mechanical process. Unlike the fuel that drives a car, hormone secretion is influenced by your reactions to external factors. If you run, you may feel your heart beating faster, and if you are startled, you might feel it lurch, but most of the time you are not aware of the way your hormones work.

During labour, your brain interprets how you feel and controls the flow of hormones to speed up or slow down contractions accordingly. Early labour can be exciting, but it can also be daunting because you know that 'this is it', there is no turning back. Most women need to get used to the sensation of contractions and the idea of labour before they can relax and submit to it fully.

As the contractions strengthen, pain warns you to move to a place that feels safe to give birth. Contractions which are strong at home often fade away when you go to hospital, however, as the different atmosphere makes you subconsciously inhibit the flow of hormones. When you feel at ease in your new surroundings the contractions build up again, but this can take quite a while. You need to feel secure for the birth process to work efficiently.

In the early stages of labour, the mechanism by which fear slows down contractions or stops them completely is not entirely understood, but being able to put labour on hold would have allowed women in hunter-gatherer tribes to hide without making any noise while a tiger passed by, for example, so it may be a survival mechanism. Today, it gives you time to reach a place where you can relax, or find someone who can give you the support you need.

Giving birth is always a momentous event for a woman. The psychologist Abraham Maslow identified it as a 'peak experience', a pinnacle in an individual's life, a single event that produces personal growth, a feeling of confidence, a blossoming of the personality.

Peak experiences are said to give life meaning, to make it worthwhile. A positive birth experience has this effect, but it is the feelings surrounding the event that produces the sense of triumph. Self-determination is a part of this.

There are as many myths about how wonderful birth can be as there are about how traumatic it can be, but you may be surprised at the reserves of strength you are able to call upon when you feel secure and empowered.

You may start labour with little confidence in your body's ability to give birth, your capacity to cope, or your power to stand up for what you want. Giving birth pushes you to your limits and beyond; when you have no option but to carry on, you gain strength as a person. A woman who tends to see herself as a frightened little rabbit often discovers that in reality she is a lioness.

The technology trap

Natural birth can take longer and hurt more than women expect, with no guarantee that it will be straightforward until after the baby is born. Understandably, in a world that likes certainty and seeks swift rewards with minimal effort, there is a temptation to intervene in the hopes of making labour easier or more predictable.

There are few absolute indications for using technology during labour and it is not always clear in advance whether it will be a help or hindrance. Technology has advantages when labour is complicated, but it does not improve the outcome when it is normal. Quite the opposite: it sometimes brings a new set of problems which can only be solved by more technology.

For some women, disruption starts with the journey to hospital and admission procedures carried out by a midwife whom they do not know. The mother lies on the bed, strapped to monitors to get a base reading of her baby's heartbeat and instead of tuning in to the rhythm of her contractions, she watches the flickering display on the machine beside her. Her midwife may be too busy to provide the encouragement she needs to get up and move around, so she stays in bed, even though she intended to be active during her labour.

Every four hours she is examined internally to establish her progress, but the hours seem long. With her partner beside her and nothing to occupy her mind she starts to wish labour away. Frustration makes the pain seem worse and when she is offered a drip to speed labour up she welcomes it. The contractions are more painful so she asks for an epidural, although she really wanted a natural birth.

Twenty per cent of first-time mothers labour slowly, gradually getting used to the sensation of contractions and releasing more hormones as they gain confidence. Such a birth can be easier to handle than a very fast labour and most women can deliver their baby successfully with patience, but they need support.

Today, slow progress is often regarded as something to avoid at all costs, but taking over and managing a normal labour can be misplaced kindness. It can separate women and midwives from their intuitive knowledge of what to do to make labour more bearable. When charts were devised to plot progress in labour, long labours came to be seen as abnormal even where there was no complication. In many hospitals, midwives set up machinery to speed up labour and to monitor the baby, but they do not offer the mother comfort or encourage her to pace herself until her contractions strengthen naturally.

When everyone expects a birth to be normal, a slow labour is not on its own seen as a reason for intervention. Routines which have little to do with safety are kept to a minimum and midwives give support freely, but where technology is seen as a saviour and midwives are accustomed to relying on it, they see reasons for using it where others might not. They are less able to judge the progress of a labour in any other way than the rate of dilatation against a chart.

Everyone is grateful when technology helps a premature baby, curtails an excessively long labour, or rescues a mother or baby in trouble; but complications sometimes arise from too little understanding of the normal birth process and inappropriate use of machinery.

An active birth is not necessarily easy, but some forms of intervention and pain relief (for example, pethidine, an epidural or a drip to speed up labour) can make it difficult or impossible to take advantage of the natural physiology of birth that has been perfected over millions of years.

Active birth

- Upright positions tend to shorten labour because gravity presses your baby's head on to your cervix (the neck of the uterus), which speeds up dilatation.
- Your uterus tilts forward with each contraction, moving with gravity if you lean forwards. This makes the contractions more effective and less painful.
- Changing position and keeping your pelvis mobile does not eliminate pain, but it makes it easier to handle and helps you to avoid drugs.
- Kneeling and squatting enlarge your pelvic cavity, giving your baby extra room.
- When you lean forward, the base of your spine swings open, enlarging your pelvic cavity by as much as 30 per cent.
- Pushing can be easier in an upright position as gravity helps, and when your pelvis is free you can arch your back to straighten the curve of the birth canal.
- If labour is slow because your baby is lying awkwardly, movement can help to shift her into a more favourable position.

Perfectly positioned

Nobody knows what influences a baby to move into the best position for birth or why some babies are more contrary than others, but when a baby is lying awkwardly the natural process of labour cannot work so efficiently. Realistically, some labours will always need help and one factor that makes a difference is the position your baby adopts in the uterus.

Babies twist and somersault like dolphins during pregnancy to help their muscles to develop; but in the last few weeks most of them line up with their mother's spine and turn head down. A baby in a favourable position fits through the pelvis more easily. The ideal position for a baby is head down with her back to your front, and her knees bent, arms crossed and chin tucked in. When a baby is well curled up like this her head matches the shape of your pelvis and her crown fits your cervix, helping to dilate it more effectively.

Around 85 per cent of babies lie with their back to their mother's side or slightly turned to her front (lateral or anterior – see Diagram 1). Place the flat of your hands on either side of your abdomen and feel gently for a firm back down one side. There may be a heaving sensation under your ribs as your baby's bottom moves, or little bumps between your opposite hip and ribs as she stretches one leg. Your baby's heartbeat will be heard low down, midway between your side and the dark line down your tummy. If her head is not engaged, you may feel it just above your pubic bone.

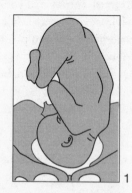

1

A baby in this position only has a short distance to rotate to the right angle to pass through the birth canal. During labour, pressure from your pubic arch can mould the baby's head into an oval shape to pass through more easily.

Babies like to be comfortable. About one in ten lies back to back (posterior – see Diagram 2), often because the placenta is on the front wall of the uterus and gets in the way. Your abdomen may look slightly flattened just below the navel and you may feel limbs over a wide area and see small bumps around your navel as the baby moves. The midwife may have difficulty feeling your baby's back and the heart will be heard at one side, between your hip bone and ribs.

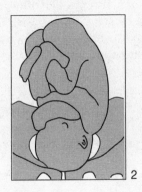

2

About one baby in two hundred lies transverse, at right angles to the mother's spine. Your abdomen will look wide and lopsided, with a hard lump resting on the flat surface of your hip bone at one side (the head) and a softer one (the bottom) at the opposite side. This is rare in a first or second pregnancy unless there is extra amniotic fluid; usually the mother has had several pregnancies and her abdominal muscles are relaxed. If your baby is persistently transverse a Caesarean section is the only option.

About one baby in seventy-five lies diagonally across the uterus (oblique). The baby's head will not be engaged (down in your pelvis) and you may feel that she is lying distinctly at an angle, from under your ribs at one side to the opposite hip. If the baby's back is towards your front you may not feel kicks; otherwise you may feel them at the top of your abdomen. Almost all oblique babies line up before labour starts.

Born bottom first

At least one baby in four is breech at week twenty-eight of pregnancy. Any time after thirty-two weeks for a first baby and thirty-four weeks for a later baby, all but 4 per cent turn head-down spontaneously. A baby sitting in your pelvis, curled up with her knees bent, is in a 'full' breech position (see Diagram 3). A few babies have their knees straight and their feet are by their ears (a 'frank' or extended breech – see Diagram 4); or one or both legs may be below their buttocks (a 'footling' breech). These positions tend to be more common in a first pregnancy because the uterus is less yielding.

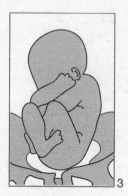 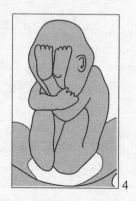

If your baby is bottom-down, the head may feel hard and round in the upper part of your uterus, underneath your ribs. It is sometimes hard to tell, however, and even an experienced midwife or obstetrician can be mistaken.

A baby born head-first can breathe straight away and once the head arrives the body usually tumbles out. A breech baby's bottom may slip through your cervix into the birth canal, stretching the muscles of your pelvic floor and making you feel the need to push before your cervix is fully open; the baby could become distressed if the delivery of the head is delayed for any reason.

Most breech babies can be born safely in the normal way if the mother's pelvis is a reasonable size, the baby is well curled up and the doctor or midwife is experienced; but you may want to encourage your baby to turn before labour.

Babies' eyesight and hearing are developed by about thirty-two weeks and they can track a light or follow a sound that catches their attention. In Germany, this has been used to encourage them to turn. The beam from a torch shines through your abdomen and the frequency of a silver chime ball (sold in Chinese shops) is easy for a baby to hear. Try shining a torch or moving a chime ball up and down close to your skin, near your baby's head to attract her attention. Then take it slowly down the side of your abdomen, shaking it all the time, in the hope that your baby will follow it round.

Traditional techniques such as crawling can be tried from thirty-four weeks, before the baby's bottom engages in your pelvis. Kneel on all fours, move your head forward, take a small 'step' with one knee, then move your opposite hand forward. Crawl 'head, knee, hand' for ten minutes twice a day in a balanced, comfortable rhythm; then lean forward with your bottom higher than your chest for ten to twenty minutes.

If you prefer, recline for ten to twenty minutes every two hours for five days, with your hips raised on pillows (so that your baby's bottom floats free of your pelvis) and your legs on a chair or beanbag. Relax and roll your hips from side to side, or put your hands on your tummy and gently stroke in the direction that feels right, willing your baby to turn.

What does it mean?

Lie: whether your baby is vertical, horizontal, or at an angle in your uterus.

Presentation: the part of the baby's body likely to be born first.

Vertex (Vx): head-down, with the baby's chin tucked on her chest.

Cephalic (Ceph): head-down, but the chin may or may not be tucked in.

Breech (Br): bottom-down.

Occipito anterior (OA): the back of the baby's head (occiput) lies towards your front.

Occipito posterior (OP): your baby's back is lying against your back.

Oblique (Ob): the baby is lying at an angle, her head under your ribs on one side and her bottom on the opposite hip bone.

Transverse (Tr): your baby is lying horizontally across your uterus.

Eng/E: your baby's head is engaged or down in your pelvis. The amount above the brim is recorded in fifths, so ⅕ means it is almost fully engaged.

NEng/NE: the baby's head has not engaged; it can be felt above your pubic bone.

Unstable lie: the baby's position keeps changing after thirty-six weeks.

Babies with attitude

If a baby is in an awkward position, labour can be long as the contractions rotate the baby or tuck her chin in; but provided your pelvis is a good size, and you are sufficiently relaxed to secrete hormones efficiently, it could still be easier than for someone whose baby is in an ideal position.

Some babies are slow to get the message that if they lined up head-down it would be easier for everyone, but they get there in the end. The best way to help your baby adopt a good position is to stay active and use forward positions where possible in the last two months of pregnancy (see Quick Guides on pages 48 and 49–50).

The head of a baby in a perfect position fits the cervix like the pointed end of an egg fits an egg cup. If the baby is lying back-to-back, the top of her head is too flat to fit perfectly and the skull bones cannot overlap or mould so well. If the baby's back is towards your front but her chin is extended her brow or face presses on the cervix, like an egg tilted in an egg cup.

No baby can be forced to adopt a favourable position, and if gentle encouragement does not persuade yours to shift there may be a reason. Some babies lie in a certain way because of the shape of your uterus or the position of your placenta and there is not a lot you can do about this, other than believe that your baby's chosen position is right for her and make the best of it.

Several factors together may make labour difficult: a baby in a poor position, a pelvis on the small side plus weak contractions, for example. Natural birth has never been the best option for everyone and if this happens to you be glad that drugs and technology are there to help you. You still have the birth you want when you change your mind in the light of circumstances.

Can birth be natural today?

From the physiological point of view, women are better able to give birth naturally today than in any past generation. They are well nourished, in better health and not worn out by repeated childbearing and rearing.

The potential for natural birth may be greater, but for various good reasons it is not easy to achieve. The society we live in views risk differently, respects those with medical expertise and relies on technology rather than intuition.

It is perfectly possible to have a natural birth in hospital, but the present culture and the attitudes of the staff sometimes make it difficult. The security some women get from knowing that technology is there 'just in case' can make it easier for them to let go and submit to their labour; but many hospitals pay no more than lip service to natural birth and resort to technology at the drop of a hat.

Giving birth is possible almost anywhere but easier in some situations than others. Contractions, controlled by the same hormones that are responsible for orgasm, can be inhibited by anxiety or disturbance; endorphins can relieve pain, but only if women are sufficiently relaxed for them to flow well. When a woman feels unsupported, her anxiety rises and her confidence in her ability to give birth falters.

If a mother knows her midwife, she does not have to adjust to new faces or answer so many questions. She is more likely to feel actively supported, not simply left to carry on so long as everything is normal. Most midwives' jobs are organised to provide constant cover for a maternity unit at the expense of continuity of care for a woman, but some women find it hard to trust a midwife they have never met.

For a woman who is sensitive to her surroundings and who is private by nature, a natural birth is easier to achieve at home. The rhythm of labour is not disrupted by travel or settling into a new environment. If she is not in labour she carries on with everyday tasks to distract herself, moving around the house instead of spending her time in a room with a bed. She may lie down to rest, but she gets up and about again, instinctively adopting positions that help the natural process.

When labour is established the midwife stays, providing encouragement and reassurance as needed. She judges progress by other signs, and may only do an internal examination if a decision involving change has to be made.

For women who want to give birth naturally, but not at home, a midwifery-led birth centre or a birth pool or a home-from-home room in hospital may provide a more sympathetic climate. Routines such as regular internal examinations, which are not essential to safety although they make running a maternity unit more efficient, can be kept to a minimum to avoid interrupting the flow of natural birth.

Technology makes childbirth safer and easier for those with a problem, but it does not help everyone. The challenge we face is to value it in the right circumstances, to regain lost confidence in women's ability to give birth, and to provide a climate in which as many women as possible can have the sort of birth they want.

In brief

- Childbirth has been perfected over millions of years. Today, women are better able to give birth naturally, if they wish, than at any other time in history.
- The delicate mechanism of birth is controlled by hormones which are affected by external factors and which flow best when you feel relaxed and supported.
- The position of the baby can affect the progress of labour. As well as dilating your cervix, contractions massage your baby into the best position to fit through your pelvis.
- Technology can help if a labour is complicated. Using it does not generally benefit women having a normal labour and it can lead to other problems.

Quick Guide: Complementary therapies to turn a baby

These therapies may help a breech or posterior baby to turn. Consult a qualified therapist if you have any concerns.

- **Acupressure:** stimulating your zhiyin points, at the outer edge of each little toe beside the nail, causes babies to move more actively, thus often helping them to turn. Press firmly on the zhiyin points with your index finger or the blunt ends of two biros for ten minutes twice a day. Up to ten treatments may be needed.
- **Homoeopathy:** to turn a breech baby, a homoeopath might suggest one dose of Pulsatilla 200 at thirty-five weeks, and a second dose two days later. For self-treatment, try one dose of Pulsatilla 30 every two hours after thirty-five weeks, over one day only, taking no more than six doses. This can be obtained over the counter from your local pharmacy. Ask the pharmacist for advice if you are unfamiliar with using homoeopathic remedies.
- **Moxibustion:** acupuncturists often recommend the slow-burning herb *moxa* or mugwort. Allow it to smoulder close to the zhiyin points, so that it warms your skin without burning you, for ten minutes twice a day for up to ten days. The levels of certain hormones change, but whether this makes the baby wriggle around or whether it is the result of all the extra movement is not known.
- **Ginger:** the Chinese claim to turn 75 per cent of breech babies after several treatments using ginger. Apply a piece of crushed root ginger to the zhiyin points every night, keeping it in place with sticking plaster. To make a paste, chop or grate the root, boil it with a little water, strain and press it through a sieve.

Quick Guide: Help your baby into a good position

If you lean forward, gravity will help your baby's spine to turn towards your front. If you lean back a great deal, your baby may slip back-to-back; and if you cross your knees, she will have no room to turn. Try to adapt these ideas if you have a disability that affects your mobility.

- **Sitting:** lean forward, tilting your pelvis with your knees wide apart and lower than your hips, to give your baby room to turn. Put two pillows on an upright chair to raise your hips, or sit reversed, leaning on a pillow. Place cushions in the small of your back when driving or relaxing in an easy chair. Use a posture chair so that your weight rests partly on your knees.
- **Standing:** keep your back straight and lean forward from the hip wherever possible, so that gravity draws your baby's spine towards your front. A sturdy box or pallet in front of the cooker or sink can help.
- **Lying down:** lie on your left side in bed, on the settee or on the floor while watching TV, so that gravity pulls your baby's spine to the left of your uterus. The shape of your uterus and arrangement of your internal organs makes a baby lying on the left less likely to turn back-to-back.

For a baby in a posterior position:
- Keep your knees lower than your hips and avoid crossing your legs.
- Kneel on the floor to read, play with your toddler, pick up toys or clean the floor.
- Kneel on a cushion, lean forward on to a chair, a space hopper, birth ball or your partner and rotate your hips for ten minutes several times a day.
- Rock rhythmically on a chair or birth ball twice a day for about half an hour.

- Make a hollow in a beanbag for your bump and lean forward on to it. This may be comfortable at night. A waterbed and swimming on your front may also help.

For a baby lying at an angle:
If your baby lies diagonally across your uterus (oblique), or her position changes frequently after thirty-six weeks, you could try this technique:

- Lie across a bath towel on your back. Put a rolled up hand towel on either side of your bump. Bring the bath towel around to hold the hand towels in place and ask someone to safety pin it quite tightly from the bottom. When you stand up the pressure may coax your baby into a vertical position.

3

Feelings and fears

No human experience is immune from fear. During pregnancy, women worry about what they eat and whether their baby is growing healthily; before giving birth they are afraid that pain will overwhelm them or that technology will be used inappropriately. Men worry about safety and what their partner may have to endure. Midwives worry about making the right decisions; doctors worry about litigation. The stakes are high and everyone cares desperately about the outcome.

Worrying is part of caring and so is not always a bad thing. It can prompt mothers to stop smoking, eat healthily and get fit, for example, and midwives to be vigilant during labour – all of which help to reduce uncertainty.

The likelihood of a healthy woman or a full-term baby coming to harm during birth is minimal compared with previous generations: for example, there are fewer than 8 maternal deaths for every 100,000 live births today, compared with around 580 in 1933. Expectations and the perception of risk have changed, however.

Fear is high on the list of things which prevent you from going for what you want in life, so it is worth putting it in perspective. It feeds on itself, mutates over time and can be unnecessarily limiting when it stems from false beliefs about yourself or about birth.

To free yourself sufficiently to have the birth you want you may need to address the issues that make you feel afraid rather than sidestepping them. You may need to change your beliefs about labour and become more aware of how risk is presented, the way you perceive it and how you respond to people whom you see as being in authority. Many of the fears that surround childbirth are associated with these.

Recognising other people's fears and facing your own is as important as any other preparations for birth; and when you take this on board you help to make your own luck.

The risk business

Boarding an aeroplane, eating out or nipping across a busy road through a gap in the traffic are chances one takes every day without giving it much thought. Birth is special, however; women invest a lot in pregnancy and care so much about the baby that, no matter how sensible they are, the whole world feels full of danger.

Risk means different things to different women, but research suggests that people are fairly predictable in how they perceive it. Unfamiliar risks and those with potentially serious outcomes tend to be overestimated. Where children are involved or the consequences of an action are delayed, anxiety is even greater.

A woman aged twenty has a relatively low chance of having a baby with Down's syndrome. Unfamiliar with the odds, she dreads the thought of any abnormality and it is several months until the birth when she would normally find out one way or the other. Her midwife points out the disadvantages of foetal abnormality tests but she decides these are acceptable: she does not expect them to apply to her and she cannot bear the thought of her baby having an abnormality.

Some people blame the media for whipping up storms about every possible hazard, but journalists are as likely as anyone else to overestimate a risk when it is unfamiliar, has potentially serious consequences and involves children. Public interest and the media reinforce each other.

Pregnant women are heavily influenced by the advice they receive from their doctor or midwife – people they see as having special trust and credibility. The concept of risk has become more important to the medical profession over the past twenty years. In theory, risk assessment should improve care because action can be planned in advance. When women are put in risk categories, however, they start to worry instead of going through pregnancy feeling special and unique. They feel that if they go against their doctor's advice or take the slightest gamble and something awful happens it will be their fault.

You may be put in an 'at risk' category, for instance, if you have previously had a Caesarean section. This means that there is merely the *potential* for a complication, not that you *have* an actual complication; and it should be a helpful reminder for your midwife. In a subtle way, however, being in an 'at risk' category can disempower you by making it harder to freely choose to have, say, a home birth or a water birth this time round.

Fear can be encouraged, consciously or not, by those who have devised ways to deal with it. Commercial interests feed the risk assessment business by determining what research is undertaken and new risks often surface when there is a product or a test that promises to lessen them. Once a 'risk' has been identified, fear feeds on itself. Anxiety is increased and it can then be reduced, at a price.

Fifty years ago women were aware of Down's syndrome but it was regarded as uncommon, especially among younger women. Amniocentesis is a test that can detect it by culturing cells from a sample of amniotic fluid (the fluid surrounding the baby), withdrawn through the abdomen. This invasive procedure was used sparingly until 1967, when the passing of the Abortion Act allowed pregnancy to be legally terminated for foetal abnormality. The Act led to an increase in amniocentesis. Women then started to worry about Down's syndrome. Less invasive screening tests were developed, but they were less accurate. False positives cause more anxiety so better tests were sought.

Pharmaceutical and medical technology firms sometimes spend large sums trying to persuade doctors of the benefits of products that address rather remote risks. Like the amulets of the Middle Ages, the value of these products lies in the feeling of security that they offer. A doctor who is impressed by a new drug or machine, however, passes on information about risks and benefits in a way that is favourable to the company. From there it is an easier (if not automatic) step to gaining the acceptance of the public.

Risk in perspective

Feelings of responsibility have a major impact in shaping your actions and they lie at the heart of the perception of risk. Influenced by your beliefs, by what other people say and by the context in which it is said, they often bear no relation to actual statistical risk.

If you are aware of how inconsistently risk can be presented you may find it easier to get your feelings in perspective. Risk is sometimes interpreted according to beliefs among researchers rather than impartial scientific standards, so one way to judge it is to view research evidence with a critical eye.

In England, women avoid soft cheeses during pregnancy because these can carry listeria, an infection that affects around one foetus in 20,000. In France, brie and camembert are widely eaten and the risk is thought too small to worry about, but women there are tested for another infection, toxoplasmosis. This affects one foetus in about 50,000; a risk considered too low for routine testing in England.

If a hundred women take the contraceptive pill exactly according to the instructions for a year, one will become pregnant. One per cent of women aged forty will have a Down's syndrome baby. For every hundred pregnant women who have an amniocentesis to detect Down's syndrome, one healthy baby will be lost as a result of the procedure. These are identical risks, but how are they judged?

The risk of getting pregnant when taking the pill correctly, or of miscarriage as a result of amniocentesis, is seen as low. Exactly the same statistical risk when applied to foetal abnormality is presented as high. Yet a woman faced with a completely unexpected pregnancy could be just as devastated as one who has a Down's syndrome child or loses a baby after a test which she chose to undergo.

You are unlikely to be warned of a high chance of getting pregnant if you take the pill, or that the amniocentesis you are about to undergo carries a high risk of miscarriage, but any woman aged forty is likely to be told that there is a high risk that her baby will have a foetal abnormality. Could there be commercial rather than logical reasons to trust drugs and technology more than women's bodies?

The prison of fear

Fear is not always rational and pregnant women are especially vulnerable to overestimating risks because they cannot bear the thought of any harm coming to their baby, let alone their being responsible for it. Nobody really expects to be the one in a million who wins the dream holiday in a prize draw; but being the one in a million whose baby has a problem seems frighteningly possible.

Everything in life carries risks, from taking a country walk to enjoying a fairground ride. You might not walk alone at night, nor take a roller-coaster ride if the equipment looks too rusty, but these activities would be less enjoyable if you focused mainly on the risks. Sometimes the things that give the most pleasure are those that other people regard as unacceptably dangerous. You personally might not choose to go hang-gliding, but plenty of people do.

Few people really want a life in which all fear is eliminated. Some of the richest experiences, including having a baby, are those which feel scary at times. Unless you are able to keep fear in perspective, your life and that of your baby may be constrained in a prison of your own making.

Every mother has to come to terms with knowing that she can only protect her child to the best of her ability before birth, during it, or in the years that follow. A totally safe existence is not all down to you, so accept fear for what it is: a valuable part of your life that helps you to make the careful and responsible choices which improve the outcome for you and your baby.

People learn and develop most when they are stretched a little beyond their comfort zone. The more their skill and judgement improve the more confident they become; they are able to undertake a greater challenge for the same level of risk.

Wherever possible judge risk for yourself, rather than relying on others who may have different agendas. You will want to rely on them when they have skills that you do not, but the level of risk then depends on their abilities not on your own and you have to trust them.

Too much anxiety can make for a pretty miserable pregnancy and birth, but you can take action yourself to reduce some risks. For example, improving your ability to recognise tension and to release it lowers the risk of being overwhelmed by contractions and of needing intervention because of this. If you are afraid of pain you could start labour using self-help techniques and add other methods of pain relief if necessary (see Quick Guides, pages 71 and 72–3).

Taking responsibility for yourself is empowering. Psychologist Karl Rogers identified the need for personal control as basic to human beings; and for many women maintaining personal control is closely related to satisfaction with labour.

A painful process

Normal labour produces normal pain, largely related to effort rather than injury. The prospect may be daunting, but any muscle that contracts as strongly as the uterus will hurt; for women who feel relaxed and supported the pain is usually bearable.

Some women genuinely believe that a natural labour will involve such agony that they prefer the major surgery of a Caesarean section. Others feel they should not have to handle pain in this day and age and that the promise of a pain-free labour far outweighs the side effects of an epidural (see pages 72–3). Many women see labour as an emotional and spiritual challenge, however. They see the pain as worthwhile and want encouragement to give them the strength to handle the challenge.

The stronger the contractions the more quickly the cervix dilates, so increasing pain usually confirms that labour is going well. If you relax and go with the sensations instead of fighting them, your body releases endorphins and enkephalins, brain chemicals that act as natural opiates and take the edge off pain.

Nobody wants pain to become unbearable, however, or to feel helpless because their resources become overwhelmed. When you want to labour naturally and have strategies to cope with pain you may need the assurance that pain relief is available just as much as those who choose to experience no pain at all.

The fear of losing control because of repeated painful contractions can make pain less bearable, so knowing that you do not have to suffer more pain than you are prepared to tolerate can take that fear away. There is no need to be a slave to pain. You can learn strategies for coping with it (see Chapter 6), or you can opt for drugs (see Quick Guide, pages 72–3).

Women who have their baby at home use less pain relief than those who labour in hospital. This may be because they are more relaxed, receive more encouragement or are more confident about their ability to give birth. Whatever the reason, it suggests that factors other than labour itself affect the level of pain a woman experiences.

In the 1940s, the great pioneer of the natural childbirth movement, Grantly Dick-Read, recognised that there is a psychological element to the way that labour pain is felt. He suggested that fear led to tension which, in turn, produced pain and that breaking the fear-tension-pain cycle through education would enable women to have a pain-free birth.

Thirty years later, Ronald Melzack, a specialist in the field of pain mechanisms, offered the theory of a neural mechanism in the spinal cord that controls the flow of pain messages to the brain. When this 'gate' closes no information gets through; as it opens more information is transmitted until messages are passed freely. The position of the gate depends on activity in the nerve fibres and on nerve impulses from the brain.

Everyday techniques for relieving pain, such as curling up with a hot water bottle for period pain, applying a cold compress to a bruised ankle, or massaging your temples for a headache, work by stimulating large nerve fibres and closing the gate so that fewer pain messages reach the brain. Changing the stimulus as soon as pain leaks through keeps the gate closed; heightened anxiety opens the gate and increases the level of pain that you experience.

Think about your attitude to pain when you decide what type of birth you want, where to have your baby and who will support you. Having pain relief because you believe that labour is so agonising that you cannot handle it is not the same as accepting it thankfully if your individual labour proves intolerably painful.

Beliefs about birth

Looking at your beliefs about birth can help to open the doors of the prison of fear. Whatever you believe affects the way you feel and act. People construct their beliefs about birth from what they see, read and hear as well as from their own experience, but each individual accepts certain things and rejects others.

Beliefs prop each other up like the branches of a rambling rose, but they do not all stand up to scrutiny or have to be taken seriously. Some are false and can be cut away like the dead wood in a rose bush without threatening the whole plant.

Every time you hear about a complicated labour (women can outdo each other describing just how awful their birth was) or someone who had a normal birth says 'I was lucky', it can reinforce a belief that labour is difficult and risky. Labour certainly can be painful or difficult, but the belief that the pain is always intolerable, or that having an easy birth is a matter of luck, does not stand up to scrutiny.

In cultures where hardship is a fact of daily life, women dislike pain but accept it as a bearable part of the process of giving birth. In developed countries, however, a remedy is sought for every problem and pain is considered something to be avoided. The experience of pain may be the same, but the perception of it and the actions taken are different.

Beliefs are made up of thoughts which create feelings which, in turn, create more thoughts; but they are just words in your head. Change a thought and you change the feeling, think differently and new possibilities open up. Doctors and midwives have acquired expertise so their advice is valuable, but the belief that you should do everything the doctor says, or that the midwife always knows what is best for you, is mistaken. Such thoughts may prevent you from considering your own preferences or from expecting to achieve them.

It can be hard to let go of habitual ways of thinking even if they do not stand up to scrutiny, but they can be changed if you persist. Like a baby learning to sleep through the night, your mind may not always give in gracefully when you question things you have hitherto accepted. It may come up with a list headed: 'But what if?' Negative thoughts such as, 'You don't really believe that, you're just pretending' may keep popping up. You may need to work at it, but once you accept that thoughts can be changed it starts to happen.

When you let go a belief that has outlived its useful life, you need to replace it with something better. Part of the challenge is to construct more realistic beliefs about birth. For most women, birth is neither wonderful nor awful, but something in between with good moments and bad ones.

Your body can handle the challenges of normal labour but if your baby is in a really awkward position you may be glad of an epidural and if your blood pressure suddenly rises you may need the help of technology. Some situations are outside your control, some fears have to be faced and accepted.

Ghosts on your shoulder

All the things you learned in childhood can hover around in your head and cast shadows over your freedom to be yourself. Think back to your childhood and the way that your parents or teachers treated you. Girls are often taught to be good, to please others; this is what gets them on in life.

Childhood patterns of behaviour can affect the way you act today, preventing you from responding in an adult way when you feel threatened. If you were greatly loved, you may have tried to merit that devotion, putting your real feelings second. If you were constantly criticised, you may have learned to conform, or to rebel. Fear can produce compliance and anger may encourage rebellion; neither of these emotions will help you to have the birth you want.

Nobody wants to be surrounded by people who criticise them all the time, but women who find it hard to accept themselves as they are sometimes do this to themselves.

Some women suppress their true feelings when an issue really matters to them, afraid that a refusal will make them lose control. They cannot allow themselves to get angry for fear of saying things that cannot be taken back, or upsetting people they will have to depend on. Expressing anger can be a safety valve, but it can also communicate how you really feel.

When you make a decision as an adult you accept the outcome. If you want a natural birth but decide to have your baby in the local high-tech maternity unit where you are more likely to end up with gadgetry and an epidural, or you are afraid that you will not be able to cope with labour and ask for a Caesarean section that is your choice. You sidestep your fears rather than deal with them, and feelings of inadequacy may still lurk in the recesses of your mind; but it misses the point to blame someone else for influencing your decision, or yourself for failing to have a natural birth. Whatever your reasons, your priorities were different.

One way to find out whether you are ready to do what it takes to get the birth you want is try to persuade your partner or a friend who is sceptical round to your way of thinking. The arguments you bring up may crystallise how you really feel as opposed to how you think you should feel.

The way you feel about birth is neither right nor wrong, so be true to your own way of thinking. Dancing to someone else's tune can set you up for failure. Why should you have a certain sort of birth because everyone else in your family did, or just because others think it is best? The challenge is to set yourself realistic goals and pay more than lip service to them; but also to be honest with yourself. Some women think they are ready to move forward when they really want someone else to take the responsibility. You cannot change other people, only yourself.

Think about what you 'could' do, not what you 'should' do, because this sets you up for success, whatever you choose. If you say 'I *could* have a natural birth if I really wanted', you can choose to do whatever is necessary to achieve it, or accept that it is a nice idea but you do not *really* want one.

Even when you know what you want the doubts may continue as the ghosts on your shoulder needle away, undermining your confidence: 'There might be a sudden complication . . . labour may be too long, too painful . . . I won't cope . . . I might fail . . . I'll make a fool of myself . . .'

You are more likely to feel empowered if you are realistic, can trust your care-givers and can express how you really feel. There may be no guarantees about who will look after you or what will happen in particular circumstances; you may have to trust that everything will be all right. You can compromise without loss of face, however: adult decisions often involve making concessions.

It is hard enough to deal with your own ghosts, without bearing those of the rest of the world as well. It is always wise to listen to advice, but you do not need to take other people's fears on board.

Other people's baggage

Relatives, friends and health professionals form their view of birth from various sources including personal experience. Their own ghosts can make them insist that their view is the right way, and can stop them from hearing what you have to say.

People with little personal experience of birth sometimes take their ideas from television, where it is rarely normal or uneventful. Drama and comedy centre on what goes wrong and how it is resolved. Birth technology looks dramatic and interesting, so the scenarios are invariably theatrical. Scenes written by people with no experience of birth and filmed at locations chosen for convenience can be unrealistic, outdated or misleading, however. It is rare to see a woman giving birth in any position other than on her back, for example.

Your partner may be concerned about your ideas or reluctant to question a professional's advice because he feels as responsible for your welfare as you feel for your baby's. Older relatives, whose children were born at a time when women did as they were told because they had no choice, may feel the natural approach worked for them and be horrified that you choose an epidural or an elective Caesarean; or they may genuinely believe that doctors know best and it is safer to follow their advice without question.

Doctors learn about labour in short bursts of drama, however, not as an unfolding process, so their view of birth can be distorted by dealing with problems. Their experience teaches them that birth is hazardous and their training teaches them to take charge, so they can find it hard when their views are not accepted.

You might wonder if female obstetricians opt to give birth by Caesarean because they know something that you do not, until you realise that they only see labours that are complicated and have little experience of the normal process. A Caesarean is a familiar procedure for them, and it largely removes that element of uncertainty. Understandably, the operation appeals to them. Like the majority of vaginal births, most Caesareans are straightforward, so a doctor may have everything to gain and nothing to lose by recommending one to his or her patients.

Midwives rarely choose a Caesarean for their own birth because they see large numbers of normal deliveries. Those who work in a high-tech environment, however, may suggest a woman has an epidural because they have neither the time nor the skills to support her through a difficult phase in her labour. Their advice may have more to do with work load, tolerance for seeing women in pain and the technology they are used to than the needs of the woman.

It is easy to be influenced by the health professionals you regard as 'experts', but their views often depend on their background. Your doctor or midwife may go by their own experience or mix of skills; a colleague may hold a different opinion and your views may also differ, without being wrong.

Today, many women have a vaginal delivery after one or more Caesarean sections, so a doctor who claims 'once a Caesarean, always a Caesarean' is outdated. Home birth is as safe for most mothers as having a baby in hospital, so a GP who implies that home birth is an irresponsible choice because there could be an emergency, is saddling you with his or her own anxieties.

Listen to advice, but judge it against the whole background, including knowledge of yourself and how you feel. Doing what you are told without thinking can give a false sense of security. You have the satisfaction of blaming other people if something does not work out, but you have to live with the consequences. Part of self-acceptance is letting go of other people's opinions or agendas.

Facing your fear

If a tiger is heading towards you, the best solution might be to hide, not to face it squarely; but if your fear is less rational than that induced by the sight of four striped legs and a savage set of teeth looking for a meal, hiding will not save you.

It is not giving birth that you have to face, it is yourself. Something within your head may make you afraid of what might happen, but there is no rule that says because you were once afraid of something you have to be afraid of it for ever, nor that what happened before will happen again. It is easier if you were helped as a child. Babies learn to fear as they grow up; if they are protected from what frightens them or ridiculed for being timid they never learn how to face fear and overcome it.

If you had a difficult first birth you may feel unable to face another labour; but by working through your fear instead of side-stepping it, you may realise that what happened was linked to unrealistic expectations, poor treatment or something that is unlikely to recur. Factors like these can be discussed and avoided by drawing up contingency plans. The right information and support may help you to come through your second labour feeling that the scars of the first have been healed; but you can find endless reasons not to do something when you are afraid.

You can tell yourself that 'they' are not likely to agree to your request so there is no point in making an issue of it. You can keep quiet to avoid upsetting a midwife or being seen as a nuisance. You can decide to tackle the issue next week, or when the right moment to mention it comes up. You can make excuses for other people: it is not the midwife's fault, she was just too busy. Your body can even collaborate with you, producing a cold or a sore throat at the crucial point.

Putting something off can prevent you from getting where you want to go, however; you hope that the problem will sort itself out and you will get what you want without making any effort. When fear is stopping you this will not happen.

If you get cross with yourself for avoidance tactics, imagine how you would treat a small child who was afraid of monsters lurking behind the curtains. Would you tell him he was silly and leave him alone in the dark, or show him there was nothing there and help him to overcome his fear? When you procrastinate through fear you are the four-year-old child who needs support to give you confidence.

Confidence has to be built on solid foundations, which also means getting enough information to enable you to share decisions. Irrational fears diminish when you are well informed and realistic. You may feel able to discard childlike dependence and share responsibility when you see your midwife's role as helping you to give birth, not managing your labour.

The people who support you can help you to feel in control. They can provide a presence in which you can use your own courage. Their love and concern for you can make the pain easier to bear; their reassurance can help you to trust your body and your intuition. They can help you to make the most of your own resources. What they cannot do is take away your anxiety, make pain evaporate or give you the courage to go on when you have no more strength.

When you successfully handle something that you were afraid of, the fear recedes and you gain inner strength. Facing fear helps to get it into perspective, although it may not banish it.

Expectations can be self-fulfilling, so positive feelings tend to generate positive results and most women need to work on their beliefs. You may have to convince your partner or family that what you want is reasonable. Doctors or midwives may be negative at first, but people who like and respect themselves tend to respect other people and they will usually help when they see you are serious.

Changing beliefs

There is nothing wrong with being trapped by your beliefs into a particular way of behaving, provided you are happy with the way things are. If not, shake off the shackles and make your own decisions. If you feel that something you were afraid of is not such a great a risk after all, change your old belief and it will lose its power to frighten you.

The first step towards having a birth experience which you can look back on with satisfaction is to become aware of mistaken or negative thoughts which get in your way and then to change them. Talk to people with different views and look at the facts (see Directory, page 215) to establish whether a belief is worth holding on to.

Write down a belief which you feel may be limiting you and identify the thoughts which reinforce it. Now change the belief and write down your new thoughts. Examples are given below:

Old belief: the doctors and midwives always know best.

Old thoughts: they are the experts; they see women giving birth every day; this is my first baby, I don't know enough about it; I should do as I'm told; they will make the right decisions.

New belief: I'm healthy and my body knows what to do.

New thoughts: I can give birth, my body knows how; people will help me; I'm not stubborn, I'll take advice if there is a complication; I'll find out enough to share decisions.

Old belief: labour pain is unbearable.

Old thoughts: I can't cope with pain; I'm not brave; I have a low pain threshold; I'll need pain relief; what if I can't have an epidural when I need it?

New belief: normal labour produces normal, not unbearable pain.

New thoughts: my pain threshold depends on how relaxed and confident I feel; good support can raise my pain threshold; I can learn how to help myself cope with pain; pain relief is available – I'll have it if I need it but I may not need it.

Old belief: the shorter the labour the better.

Old thoughts: it's taking too long, there's something wrong; I can't cope; I'll get too tired; I should dilate at the rate of one centimetre per hour.

New belief: women are not machines, some take a couple of days of regular, gentle contractions to reach three or four centimetres, then their contractions speed up and the baby arrives in a couple of hours.

New thoughts: a longer labour can be gentler; my baby needs to get into the best position for birth; I'm not afraid of a long labour, I can pace myself through it; labour will take as long as is right for me and my baby.

Old belief: women who have good births are lucky.

Old thoughts: I don't have much luck in life; I'm not good enough, or clever enough; I don't know how to help myself; they'll take over anyway.

New belief: a good birth has little to do with luck.

New thoughts: I can find the right people to help me; I can use my experience to make this birth different; I can create my own 'luck'.

More afraid than most

When you are swimming against the tide of other people's views, when a problem arises in pregnancy, when you have had a difficult birth in the past, or a very premature baby, you may feel so stressed out that you lose all sense of direction. You can tackle your beliefs, feelings of guilt, or fear of criticism, but worry tends to feed on itself unless you do something to address it. Lay your ghosts to rest.

A problem may seem to get worse before it gets better, so you need support (see Finding people to help you, page 114). Try to discuss your case with people who agree with your ideas as well as those who disagree.

You may achieve the birth you first wanted, but equally you may change your mind, reaching the same conclusions as your original advisers, but by a different route. You are likely to be more positive about the experience if you feel empowered. The end result is less important than a sense of being in control.

A previous traumatic birth

Just because your last birth was traumatic does not mean that this one will be. The past cannot be changed so you only hurt yourself by hanging on to anger or guilt. Prune away the negative thoughts so that new ones can grow and you can use what you have learned to make this birth different.

Do you still blame someone or resent them? Find a quiet place where you can be alone and bring an image of the person into your mind. Think about why they acted as they did: were they afraid of being blamed by someone else, or did their own ghosts influence them? Try to understand and let go.

If your feelings about the birth are more generalised, imagine that you are holding a large, helium-filled balloon. Draw a face on it to represent sadness, fear, anger or whatever best describes how you feel. Choose words that express the emotion as closely as possible and write them on the balloon. Then, when you are ready, let the balloon float away. Watch it disappear, taking the feelings with it.

Vaginal birth after a Caesarean

When you have another baby after a Caesarean birth you are emotionally vulnerable rather than physically at risk. Whether the operation was planned or not, subconsciously you may feel that your body failed you or that it is not up to the task of giving birth.

Morale is important in any situation where emotions are near the surface, and the feeling that you can cope with labour is more powerful than a belief that natural childbirth is best.

If you want a normal delivery, but are tempted to go for another Caesarean because you are afraid, try to imagine yourself giving birth normally, surrounded by people who will support you. Talk to people who believe that you can do it, not those who undermine your confidence or belittle you.

Focus on what you want, not on avoiding what you do not want, which tends to reinforce it. Instead of saying to yourself, 'I don't want another Caesarean birth', say things such as, 'I can have a normal birth, my body will know what to do.'

Breech baby or twins

Twins and breech babies have been born at home and in birth pools, so it is not always necessary to deliver them by Caesarean section or with high-tech care. If your doctor automatically suggests this when you prefer a vaginal delivery or low-tech care, look for another doctor who considers each case on its merits; or consider engaging an independent midwife with the necessary skills (see Finding people to help you, page 114).

Some breech and twin births carry higher than average risks, but it depends on factors such as the skill and experience of the doctor or midwife and the position of the baby or babies, so it is not the same in every case. If a doctor or midwife who is confident about delivering breech babies or twins naturally confirms that in your case a vaginal delivery or low-tech care would be risky, the advice will empower you to accept the help of technology or to choose a Caesarean birth as the best option, without the niggling fear that it might have been avoidable.

Disability

Doctors and midwives who have little or no experience of pregnant women with a particular disability sometimes overestimate the risks and constrain choice more than is necessary. Disability can cloud people's judgement so that they feel they must make decisions for you.

If you want a home birth because your house is adapted to your mobility problem, or you are used to managing your own medication, for example, your family may say you are crazy or are thinking of yourself and not your baby. Doctors may say that it would be impossible to provide adequate support for you at home.

Explore the evidence for their views and the feasibility of what you want, rather than accept one person's word. You do not have to automatically believe someone who says you are being irresponsible or that it is impossible to manage your care as you prefer. A group that advises parents with disabilities, such as DPPI (Disability, Pregnancy & Parenthood International; see website, page 217), or the self-help group for your impairment may be able to help you contact knowledgeable specialists or other mothers.

In brief

- Safety is important, but it can never be guaranteed. The way you feel about a risk may be totally disproportionate to the real danger facing you.
- You can create your own luck by analysing a situation, making

informed decisions and learning from the outcome.

- Recognise the power of your own and other people's beliefs. You may need to change the way you think about birth.
- Listen to advice, but look at the background to it and find people to help you.
- Be true to your own way of thinking, but be realistic. There is no point in crying for the moon.
- Good decisions often involve some compromise. Some fears have to be faced and accepted, but taking responsibility is empowering.

Quick Guide: Self-help for pain

Self help methods help you to handle mild to moderate pain, or severe pain for a short period. They have no side effects and you can stop using them at any time. Move from one technique to another and use them singly or in combination. For more information, see Chapter 6.

- **Positions:** stay upright, changing position from time to time; sit or kneel with your legs wide apart, leaning forward; lean on your outstretched arms, a beanbag or your partner; lie on your side.
- **Massage:** lightly stroke the skin under your bump to soothe an ache; ask your partner to press firmly on the base of your spine if you have backache.
- **Movement:** walk about, leaning on furniture or your partner during contractions; rock your body rapidly while sitting or lying down; sway slowly and rhythmically or rotate your pelvis while standing or kneeling.
- **Relaxation:** greet each contraction by blowing out gently. Concentrate on releasing tension in your shoulders, hands and jaw.
- **Visualisation:** vividly imagine a place where you feel at ease and keep your attention focused on this image, waiting passively until the contraction goes.
- **Temperature:** try a warm bath or a hot-water bottle wrapped in a towel; try a cold compress on your back, or if you are using a birth pool ask your partner to trickle cold water over your abdomen or back.
- **Breathing:** breathe slowly with more emphasis on the 'out' breath than the 'in' breath. Pause momentarily after inhaling and exhaling to keep your breathing slow.

Quick Guide: Other methods of pain relief

If self-help methods do not provide sufficient relief, TENS or gas and air can help you to handle moderate pain, or severe pain for a short period. Pethidine and epidurals help to control severe pain, but they have some side effects.

- **TENS:** a pulse is passed through four electrodes taped to your back to produce a tingling sensation. At low frequencies this releases endorphins, while at higher frequencies it blocks pain messages to your brain. Your midwife may lend you one or you can hire one (look for advertisements in the back of pregnancy magazines).
- **Gas and air (entonox):** this is a mixture of nitrous oxide and oxygen, inhaled through a mask or mouthpiece. It produces a fuzzy sensation, like too much alcohol on an empty stomach. It crosses the placenta but is thought to have minimal effect on the baby. Start inhaling at the beginning of each contraction; stop if you dislike the sensation.
- **Pethidine:** this (and meptid) is a sleep-inducing, muscle relaxant which is given by injection. Women say it distances them from pain rather than taking it away. If given too close to birth the baby may be drowsy, unresponsive and harder to breastfeed for a few days. An antidote can be given, but the baby's immature liver then has two drugs to metabolise. A 1990 study suggested that children of women who had pethidine and used entonox for more than one hour during labour were more likely to become addicted to opiates in adult life.
- **Epidural:** local anaesthetic is fed into the space around the spinal cord, close to the nerves that convey pain messages. A combination of drugs can reduce side effects and leave some sensation in your legs, but you may not get full mobility. At its best it can eliminate all pain and lower your blood pressure (useful if it is high).

You may need a catheter to empty your bladder and a drip to strengthen contractions. It raises your temperature which can affect the baby (more babies need special care) and you are three times as likely to need an assisted delivery and twice as likely to have an emergency Caesarean section. Some women complain of headaches or long-term backache.

4

Birth choices

Birth is an emotional as well as a physical experience that can be approached in different ways and that can take place in different surroundings. Some women want their baby to be born in the familiarity of their own home while others feel safer in a high-tech hospital; some feel that there should be as little intervention as possible while others reckon that if technology can eliminate pain and make labour more predictable why not take advantage of it? No single approach or place is likely to be right for everyone.

You give birth only a few times in your life so each experience should be special. You may prefer a natural approach, an active birth or a water birth, or feel more confident with foetal monitors and an epidural. You may want your labour to be actively managed or your baby to be delivered by an elective Caesarean section.

There is no such thing as the 'right' way to have a baby. Every approach has costs and benefits and your decisions depend on how you weigh up these pros and cons. If you feel comfortable and secure in your choice of where and how you have your baby it is much more likely to be a more satisfying experience.

Throughout history, claims have been made for the mystical nature of natural birth. At its best it can be an amazing and empowering experience; it can also be a long and gruelling one.

Modern technology can make birth easier and safer, but it can also give health professionals the illusion of being in control and lead to some serious problems. It is not the answer to every problem.

The best birth is the one that feels right for you, whatever that may be. The decisions are not about right versus wrong, but about respecting your own needs and about combining safety with what feels best for you as an individual.

The approach to birth goes hand in hand with where you have your baby, so you may want to consider them as a package. Most women go to hospital, although this may not be the best option if you hope to have a natural birth.

Where will your baby be born?

Home birth

This choice is open to every woman, regardless of her age, medical history, or whether it is her first baby. Your midwife brings everything that is used for a normal birth in hospital, including baby resuscitation equipment. You can get a prescription for pethidine from your GP if you think you may need it, but most women manage with gas and air, TENS, water or self-help methods of pain relief (see the Quick Guide, pages 72–3).

Once labour is established, your midwife stays throughout. You do whatever helps you to cope with labour – carry on as usual, go for a walk, have a bath, or concentrate on the contractions when you need to. Your midwife calls a colleague for back-up when you are ready to give birth and clears up after the baby arrives. You can contact her at any time and she will visit you frequently for a few days following the birth of your baby.

Midwifery unit or birth centre

This may be a large detached house or one ward of a hospital, often with a birth pool installed. It is run by community midwives, offers a similar approach to home birth, and has the same medical facilities. You would have to transfer to a hospital, however, if a problem arose or you needed an epidural.

Midwifery units are usually informal, friendly, personal and well liked by mothers who have the choice. Anyone may give birth there, regardless of age or medical history; you can also transfer from hospital post-natally for a more relaxed environment. They are not widely available, however.

Hospital

Most women give birth in hospital either because they do not realise they have a choice or because it reassures them to feel that more facilities are available, should they be needed. You are likely to have a single room for labour and birth and be transferred to a four- or six-bed ward afterwards, for a typical stay of between six hours and two days. Some women feel the atmosphere is like being back at school, while others enjoy the company of other mothers. When you return home, your midwife will visit you and help at any time is only a phone call away.

There is considerable variation between hospitals in attitudes, facilities, intervention and infection rates. If you want a natural birth, an actively managed birth or an epidural on demand choose a hospital that can offer these.

The safety issue

One would expect hospital to be a safer place to have a baby because all the facilities are there to cope with any sudden emergency. In practice, however, extensive research has shown that for a healthy mother having a baby at term (thirty-eight to forty-two weeks of pregnancy) it is just as safe to have a baby at home.

This may sound surprising until you consider that a woman in her own home is more relaxed so the natural process of birth is more likely to unfold normally. She can move around at will, making pain easier to handle than if she were lying in bed attached to machinery. She has a midwife to herself.

Very few complications occur without warning and a vigilant midwife picks up early signals that intervention might be necessary, giving plenty of time to transfer safely to hospital. Overall, about 3 per cent of babies are born with unexpected problems, most of which can be dealt with by a midwife at home or in hospital. Two per cent need intensive care, but most of these are known in advance so you would already be in hospital.

Although it is rare for a sudden crisis to arise during birth, it takes longer to get help if a woman is at home. This should make hospitals safer, but it appears to be counteracted by how they are organised. In hospital, a crisis sometimes occurs because a midwife, who often has to look after more than one woman, misses the first signs of a problem; or an inexperienced doctor intervenes inappropriately.

Technology can be misleading: the machinery can malfunction, the data can be hard to interpret. Staff who rely on technology become less aware of its drawbacks and unsafe practices can go unnoticed because when they precipitate a crisis, the equipment is there to remedy it.

At home, a midwife does not have the facilities to solve a crisis of her own making. She must always be cautious and aware, judging whether everything is normal and transferring the woman in good time if necessary.

The natural approach

Natural labour is a compelling experience where women learn about their inner strengths and find the courage to take on a new and important role. It can be intense and overwhelming, but women are designed for giving birth and using your own resources can give you the same sense of achievement that people get from running a marathon or climbing a mountain.

A natural birth starts spontaneously and, provided everything is normal, continues at its own pace without intervention until the baby is born. Your midwife relies on experience, vigilance and skilled hands rather than routine examinations. You use gas and air, TENS or self help methods such as massage for pain relief (see Chapter 6 and the Quick Guide, page 71).

In theory, you can have a natural birth anywhere, but the delicate mechanism of birth is easily upset. It can be hard to achieve in a hospital where there is lack of support or inflexible protocols that have more to do with the institution than with the physiology of labour. Even when a birth pool or a 'home-from-home' room is available, their use is sometimes discouraged because there has been 'no time to clean the room' or 'there is nobody available who can supervise a water birth'.

When technology is readily to hand, its use can become routine. Hospital staff may see the need for it where a community midwife might not, encouraging you to agree to intervention unless your labour is short. Doctors may fiddle with machinery and forget the woman wired to it, dealing with her distress by more intervention. It can be quicker for an overworked midwife to arrange an epidural than offer practical ways of coping with pain. For any or all of these reasons, you may find it easier to achieve a natural birth at home or in a midwifery unit.

Active birth

You are less likely to need pain relief or intervention if you are active rather than lying passively in bed. Most women who want a natural birth remain upright and active, especially if they are at home.

No special facilities are needed; you simply use positions which work with gravity and which help your pelvis to open during labour and delivery, as you listen to your body and respond to its signals. The positions you choose can make pain easier to handle and assist your baby in being born. Many women are too stiff to make full use of their body's versatility and need to improve their suppleness and practise various positions during pregnancy so that they can be fully active during labour.

Water birth

Water is buoyant, comforting and relaxing and you can move more freely, which makes labour easier and pain more bearable. If you like to relax in the bath or enjoy swimming, water may help you to have a natural birth. Most women can use it for at least part of their labour and its supportive action can be especially helpful if you cannot use other forms of pain relief, or if you have a Caesarean scar.

A birth pool is deeper and wider than a bath and the water is maintained at body temperature. It gives you privacy and personal space which nobody invades without an invitation and you can use gas and air and self-help methods if you need additional pain relief.

The majority of problems during labour and birth can be foreseen, and if a problem should arise you would be asked to leave the pool as a precaution. It is rare for an emergency which cannot be resolved from outside the pool to occur, although if it did the midwife would get in to help. Some women leave the water to give birth, but many decide at the last minute to stay where they are.

Water births have taken place in hospitals and homes, caravans and council flats, even out of doors. Many hospitals and midwifery units have a pool installed, or you can hire one for use at home or in hospital (see Arranging a water birth, page 91). In hospital, however, there may be rules about things such as the use of essential oils and when you can and cannot be in the pool.

Birth with technology

Most hospitals use some technology during labour, but all the evidence shows that technology does not make normal birth easier or safer. It can offer great benefits when labour is complicated, but it can also lead to unexpected problems. If you assume that it will only be used if essential, then you may be disappointed.

In many situations, using technology is an option rather than a necessity, and the amount considered necessary often depends as much on an individual hospital or midwife as on how your labour progresses.

Low-tech or mixed approach

Many women decide to start labour naturally and see how they progress. You may have no strong feelings about birth and be content to live with decisions made on your behalf; or you may hesitate to appear demanding or to make decisions you feel you know little about.

Typically, you go into hospital when your waters break or you have strong, regular contractions. A foetal monitor is attached to your abdomen for twenty minutes to get a base reading of your baby's heartbeat. You then walk around or stay in bed and a midwife pops in from time to time to check that you and the baby are fine. You are examined internally every four hours to check your progress.

If you are slow to dilate, you may be offered a drip to speed up labour and then be closely monitored because some babies become distressed if contractions are artificially strengthened. The drip and monitor remain in place until after your baby is born. Some women find it easier to lie in bed, although this is not essential.

If you choose a low-tech or mixed approach you may not get what you want automatically, so you may want to think about what is important to you in advance and tell the staff (see Birth plans, page 135). Some women say that they were swept along by a kindly midwife, or that they felt too overwhelmed by the situation to discuss anything.

Actively managed labour

Technology can be used to control labour from start to finish. Labour may either begin spontaneously or be induced and you stay in bed with a foetal monitor to record your baby's heartbeat. An epidural is inserted and you are examined internally every two hours or so.

Your cervix is expected to dilate at the rate of one centimetre per hour and, if necessary, a hormone drip is set up to achieve this. The birth is guaranteed to take place within about twelve hours, although for some women this means being delivered by Caesarean section.

You cannot change your mind once active management is set in motion, and one intervention often leads to another. Speeding labour up can distress a baby so that a Caesarean section becomes necessary. Continuous foetal monitoring may make it harder to handle pain so that you need an epidural, which makes an episiotomy (cut) and a forceps or ventouse delivery more likely.

You may accept these drawbacks, however, for the reassurance of knowing that your labour will not go on for hours, your partner will not have to watch you suffer and your baby will be continuously monitored.

Using technology in this manner has been shown to shorten the 'average' labour by less than one hour, but it can curtail a labour that would otherwise have been excessively long.

Large hospitals, teaching hospitals and private hospitals are more likely to offer active management of labour and an epidural-on-demand service, as this requires higher staffing levels and shortage of midwives already restricts its availability in some areas. Smaller hospitals rarely have the staff or the facilities.

Caesarean birth

An emergency (unplanned) Caesarean might be needed if you or your baby become distressed during labour. In most cases, 'emergency' is an overstatement: there is no great crisis and plenty of time to act calmly.

An elective (pre-arranged) Caesarean might be suggested if your baby is premature, delicate or lying in such a way that he might have difficulty negotiating your pelvis. Other medical reasons for surgery include diabetes, heart or kidney disease, extensive vaginal surgery, placental problems, fibroids, HIV, an active herpes infection or a severe form of the pregnancy-related illness pre-eclampsia.

An elective Caesarean section takes uncertainty away and it can be reassuring to know that labour will not go on for ages. You know when your baby will be born and you can plan your domestic or work commitments in advance; it is also safer than (and avoids) the possibility of operating in an emergency. Having a Caesarean sounds quick and easy compared with hours of gruelling labour, and women are said to be demanding them in ever-growing numbers.

The majority of Caesarean births are uneventful and if there is a compelling reason for the operation the advantages far outweigh the disadvantages. A Caesarean birth is not an easy option, however; when there are no complications a vaginal delivery is both safer and quicker to recover from.

The World Health Organisation claims there is no benefit to women or babies when the Caesarean rate rises above 15 per cent in developed countries. Scandinavian countries achieve this, yet the average rate in the UK is around 20 per cent and rising. In countries such as Brazil and the USA it is higher still.

This is an important issue for women. Caesareans are more expensive than vaginal births as more anaesthetists, drugs and equipment are required. More midwives are needed because women stay in hospital longer and initially they cannot look after themselves or their babies.

Unless an elective Caesarean is essential, however, you may want to consider all the implications. If you decide it is the right choice for you, it may be easier to persuade others if you have clearly thought it through and are prepared for the possible disadvantages.

Choosing a Caesarean

- The risk of death or a serious complication, although small, is four times greater than for a vaginal birth; and you are thirty times more likely to have an emergency hysterectomy for uncontrollable bleeding.
- Women report more pain after a Caesarean, around one in five picks up a wound infection and 10 per cent more babies need special care.

- You need more help afterwards as you have a baby to look after while recovering from major surgery. Breastfeeding and looking after other children may be more difficult. You cannot drive for four to six weeks.
- Studies show more post-natal depression and long-term health problems in women who have had a Caesarean birth. Around two thirds of women feel they have not fully recovered three months after the operation.
- Scar tissue in the uterus is known to reduce fertility. It also increases the risk of ectopic pregnancy (where an egg implants outside the uterus) and of placental problems in later pregnancies.
- Subsequent births are considered 'high risk' so you may have more intervention and be discouraged from having a home or water birth. There is more chance of another Caesarean, with a toddler to care for as well as a new baby.

Ask your doctor:
- Why do you recommend a Caesarean and what are the alternatives?
- What is the evidence that it is likely to be the best outcome for this problem?
- Is there general agreement, or do some doctors take a different view?

Ask yourself:
- Would having a Caesarean be worth the possible disadvantages?
- Can I cope fairly easily with a slower recovery? Can I call on extra help?
- Does the possible effect on future pregnancies concern me?

Whose choice?

Some indications for a Caesarean are clear, but there is inevitably a large grey area with little consensus. Age, treatment for infertility, a mild pregnancy complication or a distressing experience of birth the first time round may be considered sufficient reason by some doctors, but not by others.

A celebrity who has a Caesarean birth for social reasons influences attitudes in society as much as Queen Victoria's endorsement of chloroform did with respect to pain relief; and as the operation becomes more widespread it also becomes an acceptable option. One reason given for the rising Caesarean rate is that more women are choosing this sort of birth and that society supports choice.

The media typically portray women who choose a Caesarean as 'too posh to push'. This may be a neat sound-bite, but it is unfair to women. Blaming the rise in Caesarean section on 'women's choice' is too simplistic.

A woman may decide freely, but the chips are often stacked in a way that makes her 'choice' inevitable. Many women are afraid of giving birth vaginally because of a trauma they or someone close to them has experienced. If they are not offered ways that would help them to deal with their fear – continuity of care, good emotional support and a guarantee that labour will not be allowed to drag on and on, for example – a Caesarean can seem the only choice.

The way a risk is presented can sway choice, too. A woman having her first baby may hear nothing about the increased risk of hysterectomy or the effect of scar tissue on her fertility; if she has had one Caesarean she may hear about scar rupture during labour but not about the chance of a wound infection. Some doctors present a risk and leave the final decision up to the woman, who feels out of her depth: any risk involving her baby seems too great to take.

There is a marked difference in power between women and doctors when it comes to discussing birth. Women tend to be guided, so in many cases it depends on the doctor's beliefs and willingness to consider other possibilities.

It is not only women who 'choose' the Caesarean option. Doctors do not have to cope with a wound infection or care for a baby or small children while recovering from major abdominal surgery. An elective operation is safer and less stressful than operating in a crisis; it can be scheduled to fit the working day. The more Caesareans they do, the more skilled they become, but their ability to deal with certain problems in any other way diminishes, altering their perception of the risks and benefits.

In Brazil, Caesareans account for about 36 per cent of all births. A recent study[1] showed that they were performed on six times as many women who had completed secondary education and twice as many urban women, compared with uneducated, rural women. Yet 80 per cent of those who had the operation in a public hospital wanted a vaginal delivery when they entered the hospital.

The researcher investigated the decision-making process and concluded that there was no great demand for Caesarean section from women themselves, but that obstetricians were 'very active participants in the ongoing construction of the culture of Caesarean section in Brazil'.

Private care?

It is often possible to achieve something like a Caesarean section for non-medical reasons, or a home birth where your local health authority does not provide for this, but it can take effort (see Chapter 5). Some women choose private care from a consultant obstetrician or an independent midwife.

Obstetricians are qualified to conduct any labour, but have less experience of normal labour as they are generally used to dealing with complications. Friends may recommend an obstetrician, but you will need to approach your GP for a referral. If you do not know one your GP can obtain a list of those who undertake private work. The delivery could take place in a private or an NHS hospital.

---

[1] Kristine Hopkins, 'Are Brazilian women really choosing to deliver by Caesarean?', *Social Science and Medicine* vol. 51 (2000), no. 5:725–40.

Independent midwives are qualified to manage any normal labour and tend to be highly experienced at helping women to achieve a natural birth. They usually specialise in home birth, working with one or more colleagues for back-up and maintaining good relations with local hospitals. Many accept cases such as home birth after a Caesarean section. A few work in independent midwifery units or birth centres. Contact an independent midwife directly, or ask the Independent Midwives Association to send you a list.

Some independent midwives earn a modest salary and operate without insurance because the costs of this would make the care they offer prohibitively expensive. Insurance is relevant where negligence can be proved and an experienced independent midwife usually operates in a very personal and safe manner, but you may want to discuss this issue at an initial consultation.

The costs of private care vary depending on the area and the level of service you choose, but they are roughly equivalent to the cost of a good foreign holiday. If you choose an obstetrician there may be extra charges for things like your hospital stay, scans or other tests or an anaesthetist's fees for an epidural.

It may be possible to pay in instalments and costs are sometimes reduced in special circumstances.

Weighing up options

Natural approach:
- Unless there is a problem a natural approach may be better for both the mother and baby.
- If you set out to have a natural birth and either a complication arises or for some reason pain becomes unbearable, you can always add technology.
- It may be easier to have a natural birth at home or in a midwifery unit. Community midwives tend to be confident about natural birth and they are less keen to intervene.

Birth with technology:
- Technology takes some of the uncertainties out of giving birth and makes labour more predictable. It does not make birth safer for a healthy mother and baby.
- Technology can result in a waterfall effect, where one intervention leads to another that would not otherwise have been necessary. Once it is set in motion you cannot change your mind and you may get more than you bargained for.
- A mixed approach to labour means different things to different people and can cover everything from a nearly natural to an actively managed birth.

Birth at home or in a midwifery unit:
- Women tend to be more relaxed, need less pain relief, have fewer interventions and less risk of acquiring an infection at home.
- You do not, in law, have the right to demand a home birth; but equally, nobody can force you to go into hospital to have a baby. It is something of a grey area, but compromise can generally be reached by negotiation.

- There are fewer rules at a home birth: you can do as you please, anyone can be present and you do not have to leave your children.
- You have to transfer to hospital if a problem arises. This usually takes place well before a crisis situation, but emergency treatment could take longer.

Hospital birth:
- Any help needed is available immediately, but when technology is readily available it is sometimes used inappropriately.
- You may have to share a midwife with other women during labour. If the staff seem overworked, you may hesitate to ask for help after the birth.
- It can be more difficult to have a natural birth, unless your labour is short and easy. If the staff are used to relying on technology, it can be hard to hold out against it even when it is not essential in your case.
- You meet other mothers in hospital and have meals prepared for you and midwives are on hand to help care for your baby or answer questions.

Private care:
- You know who will look after you in pregnancy and labour and can build up a relationship with them. You get flexible, personal service and continuity of care.
- You can arrange antenatal checks at a place and time to suit you.
- A private hospital or midwifery unit may offer greater luxury than the NHS.
- Private care can be expensive and it is not always better than NHS care.

Shaping ideas

Having the birth you want is a progressive thought process rather than a series of supermarket choices. Some women know what they want right from the beginning, but most develop their ideas as pregnancy unfolds and they find out more about the options and what is available in their area.

If you have a pre-existing illness which could have a bearing on your labour, or if there is a real possibility that a complication might arise, you may decide to go to hospital. Otherwise, your decisions will revolve around the type of birth you prefer or the birth place which makes you feel most secure. You will have more choice if you live within easy reach of several hospitals and your health authority also provides midwifery units and a home birth service.

In the UK, a midwife is a professional in her own right and does not work under the direction of doctors, but she is employed by a local health trust that regulates her working conditions. For example, some local health authorities refuse to support home birth, and any midwife who would like to provide this choice will be putting her job in jeopardy.

If you want to give birth in hospital, but the only one in your area has a high-tech approach, it may be unrealistic to expect a natural birth. You either have to accept the likelihood of technology being used, or change your mind and have a home birth. Equally, if you want an actively managed birth or an elective Caesarean, you might have to find a hospital elsewhere to provide for your needs, or go private.

Careful preparation and good emotional support can go a long way towards making any birth a positive experience, but the decisions about where to have your baby and the approach you prefer will inevitably shape your experience.

There is a certain amount of instinct involved in knowing what is right for you, especially when your heart tells you one thing but fear overrules it. What sort of a person are you? What makes you feel secure? You need to know yourself, but also to be realistic. Take time to make the right choice.

Making the decisions

- Discuss your feelings about where to have your baby with your partner, family and midwife.
- Health professionals can give you advice but they cannot decide for you.
- Separate making the decision from the anxiety that may precede it. Review the situation in two, four or six weeks, by which time you will have made progress and realised what you really want, or decided that something is not for you.
- Do not be afraid to make a choice because it might not work out. Changing your plans might be disappointing but it is not a disaster.
- Recognise what feeds your insecurity. You will worry about things that are important to you, but you do not have to listen to people who undermine you; cut them off firmly in mid-sentence if necessary.
- If your midwife makes comments that upset or worry you, point them out. Remind her that you trust her to do her best for you and she must trust you to be realistic.
- If you are happy about where your baby will be born and the general approach to labour you can be confident and relaxed without brooding over details.

Arranging a home birth

Many doctors support home birth today, but those who still view birth as a medical emergency that is only straightforward if you are lucky, rather than as a normal life experience which throws up a problem once in a while, remain opposed to it.

You do not need your doctor's agreement to have a home birth; you can approach a midwife direct. If you do not know one, contact the supervisor of midwives at your local hospital and ask her to arrange maternity care as you intend to give birth at home. There is no need to sign any forms.

Your doctor may automatically book you into hospital, especially if it is your first baby or you are an older mother, but the choice is yours. You can change your mind at any time during pregnancy; some women need time to find out more about home birth and to decide how they feel. You may be offered an appointment with a consultant, to discuss your choice. This can be helpful, but you are not obliged gain a consultant's approval and some women prefer not to see one.

There may be a home birth support group in your area whose members offer information, lend books or birth reports, put you in touch with sympathetic midwives, or talk informally about their own experience. AIMS, the Association for Improvements in the Maternity Services, can provide you with information. Finding out the facts can reassure your partner and family, and help you to decide whether it is right for you.

If you have any problems, or you find it hard to trust your own judgement and stay determined in the face of opposition, contact AIMS.

Arranging a water birth

Be prepared to find out about water birth yourself. The encouragement you get may depend on where you live and how knowledgeable and enthusiastic your midwife is, but information is also available from libraries, bookshops, birth-pool hire companies, AIMS and the National Childbirth Trust.

Your midwife can tell you which local hospitals have a pool installed or you can check on the Internet. Bear in mind that at some hospitals one woman in five has a Caesarean section but only one in a hundred has a water birth.

You cannot usually book a hospital birth pool (someone else might be using it), but you can hire a pool for use in hospital or at home.

If you decide on a water birth at home because there are no facilities in your local hospital or you feel it would be easier, your health authority should arrange for a midwife who can supervise water births to attend you. If your midwife does not know much about it, ask her to put you in touch with a midwife in your area who does, or a mother who has had a water birth; or tell you who to contact to arrange it. Finding the right people to help (see page 114) may take some effort.

A pool usually allows a minimum of 60 cms (24 inches) of water, sufficient to cover your bump easily. You can float stretched out or brace yourself across an oval pool and some companies hire inflatables made from life-raft material which are cheaper to hire and can be filled more quickly if labour is likely to be speedy.

Pool hire companies advertise in Yellow Pages, baby magazines and the Baby Directory. Services, types of pool, prices and hire periods vary and some companies offer videos or water-birth study days, so compare prices and options.

A disposable liner, hoses to attach to the water supply, a cover to prevent heat loss and a pump for emptying the pool may be included in the fee. If your hot-water cylinder holds at least 136 litres (30 gallons), a water heater may not be necessary. The usual hire period is four weeks but you could ask about extensions or a shorter hire period; or share the cost with someone from your antenatal class.

Satisfy yourself about insurance cover and the safety of the equipment before hiring. In hospital, a pump or heater will be checked for electrical safety; at home, use a circuit breaker for extra protection. The company will give you all the practical advice you need, including guidance about where to site the pool safely.

Pools have been used in mobile homes so the floors in most houses are strong enough to take the weight. Two hundred gallons (900 litres) of water weigh roughly the same as fifteen people of about 10 stone each, so a lively party might put more pressure on your floorboards. Take account of the age of the building, the type of floor and size of pool you choose; if you have any doubts about safety, consult a structural engineer (try your local buildings inspector or Yellow Pages).

Choosing a hospital

Hospitals vary in approach and in the facilities they offer. The nearest one may offer what you want, but without information you cannot make an informed choice. Ask your midwife or GP (see Questions to ask, page 94). If necessary, phone the midwifery manager at the hospital or contact the Health Information Service for help. Compare statistical data by accessing the relevant websites.

Once you have basic information, it is worth visiting each hospital you are considering so that you can judge the atmosphere and decide if you are likely to get the sort of birth you want.

If the antenatal clinic times are not convenient, or if you have a long journey, it may be possible to attend a clinic near your work, for your midwife to visit your home, or to see your GP during evening surgery, although this may mean trading continuity of care for convenience.

Most women like to know who will care for them during labour and continuity of care is likely to be greater if midwives have their own caseload or work in small teams. Some areas offer a Domino system where a community midwife cares for you before and after the birth, and delivers your baby in hospital. Continuity can make it easier to have a natural birth. If you want this, find out the hospital protocols regarding intervention. Ask if the midwives will examine you or help to deliver your baby in any position you choose, as an indication of how flexible they are.

Very different intervention rates at nearby hospitals should be capable of explanation. Some hospitals are working towards rates of 10–15 per cent for Caesarean section, 8–10 per cent for induction, 10–15 per cent for episiotomy and 10–12 per cent for forceps and ventouse deliveries. Statistics must be interpreted with caution, but high rates at one hospital may be explained by a specialist unit, or more problem pregnancies being referred there.

Your hospital stay will be extended if there is any problem, but you may want to find out how flexible the hospital would be if you were having difficulties breastfeeding or did not feel ready to leave. A couple of days in hospital, or less, if you have a Domino delivery, can feel scary if it is your first baby, although your midwife will visit you at home and help at any time is only a phone call away.

Questions to ask

It can be daunting for hospital staff if you go in with all guns blazing, so you may want to work your questions into the conversation!

- **Continuity of care:** Where will my antenatal care take place? Are there any alternatives? Will I know the midwife who helps me give birth? Will she care for me after my baby is born? How many babies are born here every year?
- **Natural approach:** How many women have a natural birth here? Can I labour without intervention so long as my baby and I are all right? Can I be examined or give birth in whatever position feels right for me? Will the midwives give me support, encouragement and practical tips to help me achieve a natural birth?
- **Active or water birth:** Is there a birth pool or a 'home-from-home' room? Are there rules about who can use them and when? How many women had a water birth in the last month? How many had a Caesarean section?
- **Intervention:** What interventions are likely? How long would it be before my labour was speeded up? When is foetal monitoring considered necessary? What determines whether I can have an epidural? How many births are induced? How many forceps and ventouse deliveries do you do? What is the hospital's episiotomy (cut in the birth outlet) rate?

- **Actively managed approach:** Is it available at night and at weekends? Is an epidural offered on demand? Will I be induced if I want active management?
- **Caesarean birth:** How many Caesareans does the hospital perform? If the rate is high, is there a reason? How sympathetic are they to women who choose a Caesarean? What is their infection rate? What analgesia is available afterwards? How long do women stay in hospital afterwards?
- **Hospital stay:** What is the normal length of stay? How flexible will the hospital be? Will I have a single room if I have a Caesarean? Are there any amenity beds (single rooms available for a small payment after the birth)?

In brief

- Think carefully about the sort of birth that feels right for you. Try to arrange to have your baby where you feel secure and with the support of people whom you know and trust.
- Take your time to gather information (see Directory, page 215) and make decisions. You can change your mind or your booking at any time during pregnancy.
- Ask as many questions as you need to get the information you want. You can often judge by the omissions as well as the answers you are given.
- It may be easier to arrange a Caesarean birth if you can show that you have thought about and accepted the disadvantages; but if fear has prompted your choice an alternative might be to find people who can support you adequately.
- You may never feel certain that you made the right choices; just be content to do your best and get it right some of the time. You learn more if you get something wrong yourself than if other people get it wrong for you.

Quick Guide: Assistance in labour

Some labours need assistance because of a complication, but often it is the choice of the mother or midwife. You may want to find out more about the pros and cons of the help available, so that you can discuss the reason if intervention is suggested.

- **Induction:** labour may be started off if you have an illness such as pre-eclampsia (high blood pressure and protein in your urine) or if you are very overdue. Pessaries or gel are placed around your cervix to soften and thin it and your baby is continuously monitored. If labour does not start, the next step is acceleration.
- **Acceleration:** if labour is slow, your waters may be broken, using a device like a plastic crochet hook; your contractions may be strengthened with artificial hormones via a drip in your arm. Your baby will be continuously monitored.
- **Monitoring:** a foetal heart monitor can provide early warning of distress if you have a hormone drip or your baby's heartbeat is irregular. The electrodes can be attached to your abdomen by soft elastic belts, or to your baby's head via a tiny clip or suction cup. They show the baby's reaction to each contraction.
- **Forceps:** these are shaped like curved spoons and used during a contraction to assist the mother's pushing efforts. They can protect a baby's head from too rapid a delivery; or help to deliver a baby whose head is not at the best angle, who slips back between pushing contractions or whose mother is exhausted.
- **Ventouse (Vacuum Extraction):** a small metal or silicon rubber cup fits on to the baby's head and a pump extracts air over several minutes, like a child sucking the air out of a mug. Like forceps, it can help a mother who is tired, prevent a baby's head from slipping back or turn it slightly so that it fits through the mother's pelvis.

Quick Guide: Making labour easier

- A first birth is special. You may need more support, encouragement and patience than for subsequent births, where you can build on past experience.
- If your previous birth did not go well treat this birth as your first and seek out the support you need.
- Your state of mind influences your hormones which, in turn, directly affect your uterus. If you are afraid of giving birth, address this. Talk to your midwife or ask friends to suggest a good book or teacher who can give you confidence.
- If you are not happy about where your baby will be born investigate the alternatives and, if necessary, ask to change your booking.
- Learn how to relax consciously and to use your body well during pregnancy. This will help to avoid unnecessary aches and pains and will give your body the best chance of working effectively in labour.
- Ask your midwife if she could visit you at home in the early stages of labour, to reassure you and your partner that everything is going well.
- Keep the lights low if labour starts in the evening or at night. Darkness or low lighting favour your primitive brain and help you tap into instinctive behaviour.
- You can refuse any carer. If you feel upset or pressured by staff, your partner could tactfully ask the sister-in-charge if someone else may care for you.
- Sensitive support given at the right moment can raise your pain threshold and help you to cope with labour. Even if your birth partner does nothing you will value his or her presence – tenderness is more important than technique.

5

Make it happen

The key to achieving the birth you want lies in preparation. When you are first pregnant labour seems a long way off, but it takes time to change your assumptions about birth, gather the information you need to make confident decisions, or persuade others to take you seriously. Your first thoughts about the sort of birth you want may not be your last.

There will never be a 'right' way to give birth because people place importance on different objectives and their views can differ without being right or wrong. As you find out more, you may change your ideas and become open to alternatives that you had not previously considered.

It is worth checking out all the options before you assume that your choice is limited to the menu you are first offered by your doctor or midwife. Health professionals sometimes act as gate-keepers, only mentioning the options they approve of or are used to arranging. To get a variety of perspectives, read books and magazines, watch videos and speak to family and friends who have had different experiences. Look on the Internet and consult organisations such as the National Childbirth Trust.

The role of your doctor and midwife is to work with you so that as far as possible you have the birth you want. When you have gathered your information, sift out the bits that interest you, or you feel are valid and relevant. Preferences will take shape and you may be able to give yourself two or three options.

With high quality care the details of where or how you give birth become less of an issue, but there is no substitute for your own preparation if the birth is important to you. It can make you more realistic, help you to negotiate for what you want, even when it is different from what other women choose, or enable you to challenge a knee-jerk response. Above all, it can point you in the direction of people who can help and support you.

Step by step

There is a world of difference between a mad dream and an achievable ambition; whatever your aim, you need to know what you want and why you want it. Share your thoughts with other people so that you always have some back-up and stick to your guns without allowing yourself to be sidelined or distracted by someone else's agenda. Success is more likely if you believe that your goal is achievable and plan in realistic steps.

In a nutshell, decide your goal, look at what you have achieved and what still needs to be done, recognise what is stopping you, give yourself credit for your strengths, and identify the changes you need to make in order to achieve your goal.

Step 1: Identify your goal

You can only make goals for yourself, not for other people. Work out what you want and express it as something positive: for example, 'I want an epidural on demand', instead of 'I'm not going to be left in pain for hours like last time', or 'I want to have a natural birth', rather than 'I don't want any drugs or intervention.'

Phrasing your goal in a positive way is more constructive. Leave out the 'if it goes all right' or 'if possible': they may indicate flexibility to you but uncertainty to other people. You can change your plans (see Changing your mind, page 168), but you may be taken less seriously if you seem ambivalent from the start.

Whether your choice is instinctive or the result of much deliberation, clarify your reasons so that it will be easier to persuade others should this be necessary. To feel confident and get other people's support, you need to be sure that what you want is safe, reasonable and achievable. Talk to other people who have achieved it (see Finding people to help you, page 114). Do some research so that if someone opposes your choice you will know enough to judge whether they have good reasons for doing so, or are simply trotting out a personal opinion dressed in the cloak of fear or the hat of authority.

With lateral thinking, creative solutions often present themselves. The London tube map shows how the stations are linked, not where they actually are in relation to one another. For tube travellers this is more useful than a real map because the key question is not 'where is station x?', but 'how do I get to station x?'.

Your key question, once you have identified your goal, is not 'Will I be allowed to do this?', but 'How do I achieve it?' When you are clear about what you want and people can see you have thought it through, even those who are initially opposed or indifferent often rally round.

Step 2: Check your progress

Make as complete a list as possible of everything that needs to be done to achieve your objective. Run it past your partner or a friend to see if there is anything you have forgotten. Cross off anything you have already done and put the rest in a rough order. You will now have a clear picture of what you have achieved so far and what still needs to be done (see Progress lists, opposite).

Few goals are attained in one giant leap. Most are reached by a series of baby steps or intermediate actions. These may include gathering information, confronting fears and changing your beliefs, or finding the people who can help you and bringing family members or health professionals on board. Persuading people can take longer than collecting basic information, but the blocks will gradually fall into place, building a staircase to reach your goal.

Progress lists

Gina's mother, her partner Dave and her midwife are not keen on a home birth as it is her first labour, but her cousin Lucy had her first baby at home and Gina is sure this is what she wants. She needs everyone to feel comfortable about her choice, but she also wants to be seen as reasonable.

- Get more information, including research evidence on safety, to boost my confidence and reassure Dave and Mum.
- Invite Lucy and Martin for supper to tell us their experience (ask Mum over?).
- Is there a home birth group in this area? (I need support and useful contacts.)
- Work on assertiveness: I am not being unreasonable or difficult in wanting a home birth.
- Talk to midwife again. Reassure her that it's not a whim, I've thought it through and accept that I might need to be transferred to hospital etc. If still negative, ask if she knows anyone else who could help.
- Find a supportive midwife (contacts from home birth group?) and ask her to meet Dave and Mum to help reassure them.

Maxine's first baby was born in her local hospital and she could not have an epidural because the only anaesthetist had been called away to cover an emergency. She is determined to have one this time round.

- Find other hospitals in this area offering twenty-four-hour epidurals (check information on Internet).
- Check their other facilities, convenience, distance etc. and make appointments to visit them (in order of preference).

- Write down questions to ask. Are there circumstances when they could not offer an epidural on demand, eg. only one anaesthetist on at night, labour ward closed for staffing reasons so new arrivals sent to another hospital?
- If hospitals near here cannot guarantee me an epidural, see if there is one near Mum's house and discuss staying with her.
- Possibly consider private care (check cost – could we afford it?).

Step 3: Overcome obstacles

What stands in your way of achieving your objective? Sometimes what appears to be a barrier put up by someone else is in fact one of your own making.

The pathway to any goal is rarely straight and smooth; there are usually hurdles which you could not see at the start, which at first look insurmountable. When you look at them objectively, however, you may see ways round them.

If your family does not support your preference because they are anxious, could you find the people or information to reassure them that your choice is safe (see Finding people to help you, page 114)? If the consultant at your local hospital does not support your reasons for wanting an elective Caesarean, could you travel further afield? What is stopping you?

If your health authority does not provide a home birth service, you could work on your assertiveness skills (see page 120) and persuade them to fund some or all of your care from an independent midwife; or pay for one yourself by taking out a loan, asking a relative for help or asking to pay in instalments. You could arrange to have your baby in an area that does offer a home birth service.

All these strategies take extra effort and sometimes the only solution is to set aside your original goal for the time being. It may be that you have neither the time nor the energy to do what is necessary to achieve your original goal at this point in time. Circumstance is a valid reason for modifying a goal when you cannot reduce your commitments or ask your partner, family or friends to help.

Sometimes circumstances are outside your control. Your heart might want a natural birth, but if a Caesarean section is safest and you accept this, there is no point in getting upset. You can choose to redefine your goal because your overall priority is your baby's welfare; a new aspiration might be to achieve a Caesarean birth that you feel good about (see Birth plans, page 135).

When you keep your eyes on your goal, you are less likely to see the obstacles in your path as insurmountable; but if you cannot achieve all that you want, settle for a compromise. Compromise is not failure. You can still feel empowered if you make the decision.

Step 4: Recognise your strengths

Motivation provides the mental bridge between thoughts and actions. By analysing your strengths and recognising your assets, you may see new ways to get round obstacles. Everyone has abilities that help them to achieve their goals.

Write down your strengths and your assets. At first, your mind is likely to go completely blank, but gradually you may start to recognise character traits and attributes which can help you to achieve your goal. Ask other people what they think are your strengths – they may see qualities which you take for granted.

Take your time; this is an ongoing exercise, not a rainy day diversion. You may find yourself adding to the list over several weeks and the more strengths and assets you recognise the better. Any one of them may point the way to a new line of thought, or give you the confidence to tackle a hurdle.

A list recognising your strengths and assets can help if you are afraid to commit to an idea and decide not to try because failure would be too demoralising. Knowing what you want and not pursuing it for fear of disappointment misses an opportunity to get something positive out of an experience.

Strengths and assets

Gina: I generally get on well with people; I can take responsibility for myself and my life; I'm willing to change; I'm interested in finding out more about birth; my family and friends care about me; I can usually find some common ground to defuse an argument; I have achieved other goals and am motivated to achieve this; I can listen to advice, but make my own mind up; I'm sensitive to other people.

Maxine: I can be assertive without being aggressive; I persevere when I want to achieve something; I am fairly organised and can plan well; I enjoy doing research if something interests me; I can count on my partner's support; I'm optimistic; my decisions generally turn out to be right; when I know what I want I'm pretty determined; I see most things in a positive light.

Step 5: Make changes

An awareness of your strengths and assets may help you to make any changes necessary to reach your goal. Beliefs are a common stumbling block. You may have to address fears about birth and pain, or become more confident about your body's ability to give birth to a baby safely. You may have to adjust your perception of risk, decide that a risk is worth taking, and accept responsibility for the outcome. It is easy to complain when you do not get what you want, but sometimes the responsibility lies in yourself.

If you have no problem in being assertive in your job, but find it hard to ask for anything for yourself, you can learn to separate your own needs from what you assume your family expect you to do, so that you can act independently. You can learn to speak to health professionals on equal terms and challenge them with research evidence if they put forward their personal views as the 'right' ones.

It may be necessary to carve out time to focus on the birth by adjusting your lifestyle, or to persuade your partner to change his so that you have time to focus on the birth together and you feel able to rely on his support. You cannot force other people to do what you want, but when you act differently their response may also change.

People may be more understanding about what you want if you explain why you have chosen it. A hospital with a standard procedure may be willing to compromise if you persist politely. A midwife who tries to put you off having a home birth may change her attitude when she realises you are well-informed and not in pursuit of some romantic fantasy.

These are all achievable changes. They demand effort on your part, but when you set your mind to it you may be surprised at the progress you make. Change embraces the possibility of failure and can be daunting, but it is also an opportunity to learn more about yourself.

Effective care

In the eighteenth century, disagreement between doctors and midwives centred around who was in charge. There can be turf wars between midwifery and obstetric approaches today and in some areas a similar conflict exists, albeit in a restrained way, between health professionals and parents.

Effective care has to be achieved by agreement. It may never be possible to have a completely free choice as resources will always be restricted, but neither a health professional nor a woman can insist on a particular course of action.

Doctors and midwives can recommend something and provide evidence of its benefits, but they cannot save you from yourself or from making what they consider to be the wrong decision; nor can you insist that a health professional treats you in a particular way or place. Where there is disagreement, however, the relationship should be one of equals seeking the best solution, not one person dictating what the other is allowed or obliged to do.

A doctor will be influenced by the medical aspects of your pregnancy and birth, but for you there will also be social and psychological factors pulling you in different directions. The priority you attach to the various factors will differ from your doctor's priorities and, unless these differences are taken into account, you are less likely to receive satisfactory care.

When someone designs your kitchen, they advise you about safety, about the placing of the units, and will come up with various options about what it could look like. Building regulations and the position of the water, electricity or gas supplies affect the design, but most elements are a matter of preference. You may know exactly what you want at the outset or deciding may be a gradual process. In an effective partnership, however, you will end up with the right kitchen for you.

Your final kitchen design may or may not reflect the designer's personal taste, but you are the one who has to live with it; just as you are the one who lives with the consequences of choices made about birth.

In the same way, a doctor or midwife should give you advice about safety and the overall benefit of their experience, but they should not impose their preferences on you. Health professionals do things *with* pregnant women today, not *to* them. A parent–child interaction is not the relationship of people working on the same level to make the best decision in the circumstances.

Taking control away from women, except in a genuine emergency, can contribute to the culture of blame in obstetrics. A woman who is treated like a dependent child may overreact to protect herself. If a decision taken over her head turns out badly, she may be incredibly angry, even when the action was well-meant.

If you want to share important decisions, however, you will need to find out as much as possible during your pregnancy. Ask questions when there is something that you do not understand. Listen carefully to advice because in many situations you will want to follow it; but make your own decisions. That is your right.

Effective care depends on communication and creating a dialogue of mutual understanding that leads to shared responsibility for decisions. It takes a conscious effort on both sides, but it can build trust and allow you to stay in charge of your own life to the degree you want.

Creating a dialogue

In a classic psychological experiment using hidden cameras, people were politely asked to give up their seat on a train. Fifty per cent of them agreed. As there were plenty of spare seats it could be said that they had no reason to refuse: the consequences were not to their disadvantage. When the person asking was accompanied by someone in a uniform, however, every single person complied!

This may have something to do with subconscious feelings about authority figures. Something similar happens to many women when they are talking to health professionals. They feel quite unable to challenge ill-informed opposition, or tackle a 'doctor knows best' attitude.

There is no reason why a healthy woman going through the most normal of female life experiences, a woman who in any other situation would ask questions and make her own decisions, should accept the judgement of a doctor or midwife without hesitation and feel that she has no option but to comply. You may want to trust the experts and they may be sure of their judgement, but health professionals can make mistakes or hold beliefs which are outdated, just like anyone else.

Nobody wants to base decisions on information that is out of date or on views that are biased, so research evidence is a useful part of any dialogue. Research is intended to ensure that any treatment offered, or procedure carried out, is effective and of overall benefit to patients. It can resolve differences of opinion, enable your doctor or midwife to provide an alternative you prefer, or help you to accept that a course of action is justified. The aim is discussion, not confrontation.

You do not have to become an expert in your own right, but it is easier to have a true dialogue if you can ask appropriate questions. Knowing your facts strengthens your sense of being equal and can give you the confidence to ask for a second opinion if necessary.

Some health professionals are unaware of how subtly they take control of women's choices, especially in hospital, where it tends to be part of the culture. A woman who asks questions may be made to feel that she does not know what she is talking about, so that her confidence crumbles and her autonomy flies away.

Others find it hard to accept that informed consent goes hand in hand with informed refusal. They assume that a woman who rejects advice has not understood the situation when in fact she may have understood perfectly, but simply have a different perception of risk, or decide against it for her own reasons.

If you meet with opposition, allow time for reflection before revisiting the subject; an initial refusal may not be the final word. Some women like to get things down in writing, but through dialogue you may change the other person's mind or they may change yours.

Inner strength

Acting assertively is easier when you believe that you have a right to be treated as an equal human being. You build your sense of inner strength by respecting your own needs, feelings and rights while equally respecting those of other people. If you can recognise and identify your feelings, accept them and express them appropriately, you are well on the way to being your own woman.

Confidence can be fragile when you are heavily pregnant, thinking of your baby as well as yourself or facing someone wearing a frown and a stethoscope. Many women are perfectly able to take responsibility or act in a reasonable manner when their own welfare is at stake, but not when it involves their baby; and this shows in their manner and their body language.

Body language emerges from your inner feelings and it can reinforce or cancel out what you are trying to say. If your tone of voice, facial expression or posture indicate doubt or uncertainty these non-verbal messages may speak louder than words. Some women fail to get what they want because they overreact when they feel

Asking questions

Think about what you want to know and work your questions into the conversation – firing them off in quick succession can appear aggressive!

- Why do you recommend this treatment (procedure, approach)? Could you summarise the evidence? (If not, check for yourself – see Directory, page 215.)
- What are the advantages and disadvantages? Are there any other disadvantages? (Prompt in case some have been forgotten.)
- Is this treatment essential or just one option? Can we discuss other options?
- Are there differences of opinion between experts?
- What is the success rate for this treatment? How do your outcomes compare with those of others in the field? (A delicate question needing an open answer.)
- Is it safe for the baby if I do this? Is it safe if I don't do that?
- Could my partner and I have a second opinion?
- I am not sure about this treatment (procedure). May I have more information?
- Unless it's urgent we'd like some time to consider it. Could we think about what you have said and talk to you again? (Gives time to check alternatives.)

threatened, and push their own point of view, ignoring anyone else's. Less forceful personalities drop hints, but get upset when other people do not pick them up; or they opt out, leaving others to take decisions for them.

Aggressive, manipulative or passive behaviour tends to make others feel defensive or guilty and, in response, they take control. They may try to make you feel ignorant to bolster their authority, or imply that you are being selfish, foolish or the odd one out when everyone else accepts the status quo.

Many women find it hard to confront people they see as being in authority, even when they are certain of their ground. Being different does not mean one is unreasonable or irresponsible, but disapproval or rejection is an uncomfortable feeling and it can hit at the roots of self-esteem, sowing the seeds of self-doubt.

An assertive woman does not automatically get what she wants, but she is not over-dependent on the approval of others, and so when a request is refused she does not feel totally demolished. She knows that everyone has negative as well as positive qualities, recognises her own needs and is able to ask openly for them. Her inner strength means she expects to be treated as an equal.

Look at the list you compiled to monitor your progress (see pages 101–2) and select the situations which you would like to handle more assertively. Write down next to each how you would deal with it at present, without attaching any self-criticism to it. Your aim is to be more aware of how you normally deal with a situation, so that you can decide to change aggressive, manipulative or passive behaviour.

Starting with the scenario you find easiest, so that when you try it out and succeed you will be encouraged to tackle something more difficult, consider how you might deal with each situation assertively (see Quick Guide, page 120).

Politely persistent

Most health professionals prefer to be helpful if they can and have no desire to be obstructive. It is better to get a result by polite persistence than to resort to aggressive, manipulative or passive tactics, as the following examples show.

Pauline's goal: to arrange an elective Caesarean section

Pauline: 'Could we discuss having a Caesarean section, please?'
Midwife: 'Oh, you won't need one unless there's a complication.' (deflection)

Knee-jerk reactions

In some areas, elective Caesarean section or home birth elicit an automatic refusal. Use your assertiveness skills to field knee-jerk responses.

'You cannot have a Caesarean birth because . . .'
'You're a healthy young woman, you don't need major surgery.'
My past experience (explain) suggests it would be more damaging psychologically for me to have a normal birth. What emotional help will you provide to help me cope both before the birth and afterwards?
'It carries higher risks and recovery takes longer.'
I understand and accept this, but elective Caesareans are very safe. I have thought this through and organised extra help for afterwards.

'You cannot have a home birth because . . .'
'I've seen people bleed to death at a home birth.'
That must have been frightening for you but it doesn't mean that I will bleed to death. How often does a serious haemorrhage happen? If a problem arises I can be given intravenous syntometrine or transferred immediately to hospital.
'We have no staff available.'
How often does that happen? What happens when you are short of staff in hospital? What is your home birth rate? (Are they meeting the demand in the area?)
'We don't have a flying squad in this area.'
The ambulance service transfers women quickly to hospital elsewhere – is it a problem in this area?
'There is no demand for home birth in this area.'
How do they know? What research has been done to check the demand? Could I see the results?

P: 'I'd really like to talk about it.' (broken record)

Mw: 'You're only twelve weeks pregnant, we'll talk about it later on.' (deflection)

P: 'I want to know how I can arrange to have one. Could we discuss it today?'

Mw: 'Giving birth is perfectly normal, you know. There's no need to be afraid.'

P: 'I know it's normal, but it's not right for me. I have always known that if I ever had a baby I would need to discuss an elective Caesarean early in my pregnancy.'

Mw: 'It's not an easy option and I don't think the consultant will agree. The health service can't afford to offer a Caesarean to anyone who wants it.' (deflection)

P: 'It's not a whim. I'm just not able to handle a normal birth because of something in my past. I really want to know about a Caesarean, please.' (broken record)

Mw: 'Ah, I see. In that case of course we'll talk about it today.' (a result!)

Sara's goal: to change her booking from consultant unit to midwifery unit

Sara: 'I'd like to change my booking from the consultant unit to the midwifery unit.'

Doctor: 'You're thirty-seven weeks, aren't you? It's rather late, don't you think?' (deflection)

S: 'Yes, I'm thirty-seven weeks. Could you arrange it, please?' (broken record)

Dr: 'Have you visited the main unit? It's really nice, you know.' (deflection)

S: 'I've looked at both and I'd like to change my booking to the midwifery unit.'

Dr: 'Why do you want to change? They've got all the equipment in the main unit if there's a complication. You don't know what sort of labour you'll have and transferring in the middle of labour could be stressful.' (deflection)

S: 'I know, but I've decided that I want to give birth in the midwifery unit.'

Dr: 'I'd have my first baby in the main unit, if I were you.' (deflection)

S: 'Lots of women prefer it, but I'd like to change to the midwifery unit, please.'

Dr: 'All right, if you're sure that's what you want.' (a result!)

Lizzie's goal: to speak to her own midwife

Lizzie (phoning): 'I think my labour has started. Could I speak to my midwife, Maggie, please?'

Midwife: 'Maggie's busy at the moment and we're short staffed this evening. I'm afraid you'll have to come into hospital to have your baby.' (deflection)

L: 'But I've booked a home birth. Do you mean I can't have my baby at home?'

Mw: 'We're rushed off our feet. It might put other women at risk if Maggie goes off to a home birth. You wouldn't want to put babies at risk, would you?' (deflection)

L: 'I discussed this with Maggie. She said that if you were under-staffed you would get someone from the midwives' bank. Could I speak to her?' (broken record)

Mw: 'I suppose we could use the bank, but it would really help us if you came in. (pause) . . . I'll call Maggie, if you insist.'

L: 'Thanks, I'd really like to talk to her.' (broken record)

Mw: 'You're lucky, she's just come in. I'll hand you over.' (a result!)

Julie and Steve's goal: to use the hospital's birth pool

Julie (arriving at the hospital): 'Could we use the pool room, please?'

Midwife: 'I'm not sure if it's free. Stay in this room for the moment.' (deflection)

J (when midwife returns): 'Is the pool room free? I'd like to use it.' (broken record)

Mw: 'There's nobody in it but we haven't had time to clean it properly.' (deflection)

J: 'Could somebody do that because I really want a water birth.' (broken record)

Mw: 'I haven't been trained to supervise water births.' (deflection)

J (feeling desperate): 'Is there anyone else? I really want to use the pool.'

Mw: 'We're a bit short-staffed tonight.' (deflection)

Steve: 'This is something that's important to Julie. We'd really appreciate it if you can get the pool room sorted so that we can all make this birth good for her.'

Mw: 'Yes, of course. Let's get you settled in there and I'll clean the pool myself. Jan has done the water birth training course, she'll look after you.' (a result!)

Finding people to help you

When you are unable to have the sort of birth you want because a problem arises, it is disappointing, but easier to come to terms with if you are satisfied that the change of plan is necessary for your own or your baby's welfare. This is a case of making a different choice because the circumstances have altered.

When the system or someone in it denies you a choice that is important to you, or you are told that something considered reasonable elsewhere is not available for you, however, it can be harder to accept. The tide of fashion may be running against you, or morale among local health professionals may be at such a low ebb that the extra effort required to provide what you want is lacking.

Some health authorities think they know what is best for mothers and they see no need to cater for a variety of approaches. They draw up choices and strategies before consulting anyone, then devise ways of appearing to listen to women's views before telling them what is good for them.

Facing stone-wall opposition is especially hard when you are heavily pregnant and the birth is a fast-looming deadline. If you meet with constant hostility you may veer from being certain that your choice is right and that getting it is worth the effort, to not caring what sort of birth you have and just wanting it to be over because the stress is all too much.

Achieving the birth you want often depends on finding the right person to help you. Most women who are facing opposition feel vulnerable and need people to share experiences, provide unbiased information or give emotional support. Friends, work colleagues, a sympathetic midwife, voluntary organisations such as the relevant disability group, the National Childbirth Trust, or AIMS, may be able to put you in touch with the right person locally. A network of women of all ages and persuasions, for whom the birth experience is important in its own right, helps others by providing contacts or answering specific queries.

Out there somewhere is the support you need. Set yourself a realistic deadline and enlist the help of everyone you can. Try to keep the energy positive, and your goal as clear as possible. Keep your story simple: you may be passed from person to person until you find the one who can help you. Get on to the grapevine and exercise patience.

Keep a diary

Brief notes about what happens, when it happens, and how you feel about it, helps you to keep track of your progress and they make a useful record to look back on.

Petrina's Diary

Petrina and Martin live in an isolated area and are expecting their first baby in October at St Catherine's, their nearest hospital.

26 March: Antenatal at St Catherine's, 2 p.m. A long journey and a long wait. They seemed very rushed and impersonal. No chance to ask questions.
21 May: Anomaly scan, St Catherine's, 10.30 a.m. Short wait but staff were very busy. Didn't like to bother them with questions.

Seems like a baby factory. Not sure I want to give birth there!

26 May: No midwifery unit locally and they don't do home births – everyone goes to St Catherine's. Martin pointed out that the labour ward may be different from the antenatal clinic, so we've arranged to go on a tour.

16 July: Tour of labour ward, 4 p.m. Confirmed my fears. Kindly, but overworked staff who told me what I would and would not be allowed to do!

18 July: Martin checked Internet for a midwifery unit near Mum so that I could stay with her, but no luck. He suggests a home birth, although the midwife said they don't do them. Getting anxious – only ten weeks to go and I want it sorted.

30 July: Antenatal check, 3 p.m. No home birth service – maternity services 'centralised on grounds of safety and cost'. Martin wants to challenge this.

31 July: I agree it's wrong to concentrate resources on one kind of care, but I feel low. Phoned the National Childbirth Trust for support and contacts. They say the government expects health authorities to offer choice and there is no evidence to justify refusing home birth on the grounds of cost or safety. Martin has written asking the health authority to reconsider.

1 August: Contacted the Independent Midwives Association. No independent midwife close by, but after we had talked, Alison was prepared to travel to discuss my birth. Boost to morale.

13 August: Health authority replied that their midwives have no experience of home birth, but without attending them midwives won't feel confident and unless they feel confident they won't attend! Someone has to break the cycle. Phoned to set up a meeting with HA. Fed up – this seems to be endless.

15 August: Meeting with independent midwife, 7 p.m. Felt really confident with Alison. If we can't negotiate a compromise with the health authority (meeting on 1 Sept – I'm dreading it), we've decided to take out a loan to pay for her care.

1 September: Health authority meeting, 10 a.m. Martin took a day off. We asked them to pay Alison's fee because they cannot provide me with choice. After much discussion they agreed it was in their interests to tackle this issue and will pay part of the fee. My midwife will attend to build up her skills. Feeling brilliant!

5 October: 6 a.m. Harry was born at home and it was beautiful. We didn't even consider this as an option until July, but people were willing to help us.

Marie's Diary

Marie and Doug have five-year-old twins and their baby is due in early January.

7 December: Antenatal check, home, 11 a.m. Baby is breech. Midwife says four out of five turn before labour and some breech babies can be repositioned by external version.[2] Otherwise, I'll need a Caesarean. No driving for six weeks – how will I cope? Doug has a work trip to Canada in February.

14 December: Antenatal check, St Anselm's, 10.30 a.m. Baby still breech and another midwife said the consultants at St Anselm's have no experience of external version so if the baby doesn't turn, I'll need a Caesarean. Felt devastated. Phoned the AIMS for advice and they say there's a consultant at Walton Edge who may agree to try and turn the baby.

28 December: Consultant appointment, St Anselm's, 11.30 a.m. Still no change. If the baby remains breech, the consultant said an elective Caesarean will be best all round, but when pressed he referred me to Walton Edge hospital for external version. Doug has postponed his Canada trip.

3 January: I have transferred my booking from St Anselm's. The consultant at Walton Edge was lovely. She asked me to come in as soon as I feel mild contractions and we'll make the decision then.

9 January: The consultant turned the baby. It was a bit uncomfortable but my contractions strengthened almost immediately and Hannah was born in four hours. I'm so glad it was a normal birth. I feel brilliant!

---

[2] See box, page 118.

External cephalic version (ECV)

Research has shown that turning a baby in a breech or transverse position is effective in about 70 per cent of cases, reducing unnecessary Caesarean sections. After a scan to determine your baby's exact position, the doctor gently manipulates her through your abdominal wall. It generally takes about half an hour and may be uncomfortable, but not painful.

Success depends on the skill of the doctor, the amount of amniotic fluid, and whether you have already had a child – if so, your abdominal muscles are likely to be more pliable. External version is more likely to succeed if your baby's head is easy to feel, her bottom is not engaged, and your uterus is relaxed (you may be offered a muscle-relaxing drug), but if the first attempt fails you may be able to try again.

In brief

- Preparation and forward planning are as necessary to achieving the birth you want as they are for any other important occasion in life.
- Recognise your strengths and make the changes you need to in order to achieve your goal.
- Expect to be treated as an equal. If necessary, work on your assertiveness.
- Opposition can make you feel very vulnerable. Find people to support you.
- The certainties in any situation change over time so flexibility is a genuine asset.
- If you build steadily and make each action count, everything will suddenly fall into place. People will help you (see Directory, page 215, for addresses and websites), but nobody can achieve your goal for you.

Quick Guide: Affirm your rights

It helps to remind yourself of something easily forgotten when you are under pressure – your human rights. These include the right to:

- State your needs and set your priorities without having to justify them.
- Be treated with respect as a capable and equal human being who is not stupid, ignorant or irresponsible.
- Express your feelings, opinions and values. If they differ from everyone else's, it is a matter of perception, not of right or wrong.
- Give informed consent or informed refusal when offered any procedure or treatment, without giving a reason.
- Say when you do not understand something. Needing more explanation does not make you a stupid person.
- Ask for what you want and change your mind at any time.
- Make mistakes. A wrong decision does not mean you are a foolish person; not following orders does not mean that you are selfish or irresponsible.
- Leave other people to address their own problems or fears.

Quick Guide: Assertiveness techniques

Assertive people tend to use three classic techniques:

Decide what you want or feel and express it specifically and directly.
Directness is perfectly courteous when offered in a relaxed and friendly way and getting straight to the point is extremely effective. Hints which seem perfectly obvious to you may mystify everyone else; if you beat about the bush, people may misinterpret your needs. Make a clear, unambiguous request at the outset. You only weaken your point and confuse your listener by padding your statement with anxiety-led additions such as 'I don't know how you'll feel about this . . .' or 'Maybe it isn't possible in my case, but . . .'

Repeat your statement over and over again if necessary.
Acting assertively means maintaining your confidence and keeping your goal in mind despite any anxiety you may feel. If your wishes or concerns are dismissed, keep calm and keep going. When you have said what you want, repeat it patiently like a broken record, even if your listener raises irrelevant arguments in an attempt to deflect what you are saying.

Field responses which undermine your position.
If you are well-prepared and have the facts at your fingertips, you can handle a situation that you might otherwise find so intimidating that you back down immediately. Fielding responses is part of any discussion between equals and, on a practical level, it avoids being crushed by negative or dismissive comments. By remaining confident and keeping up the dialogue despite deflections, it is often possible to find ways around an obstacle, or a solution that satisfies everyone.

6

Ready for birth

Giving birth can be an overwhelming experience, with all the excitement and fear which this implies. Few women are dealt a perfect labour and few have all the cards stacked against them. Most births are somewhere in between, harder than unzipping a banana but not nearly as tricky as opening an orange.

You do not have to behave according to rules, nor expect higher standards of yourself than you would of other people: a good birth has nothing to do with whether you labour naturally or use technology; nor is it linked to feeling little or no pain. It depends to a large extent on what is important to you and whether you are able to handle the experience in a way that makes you feel capable and positive.

How you choose to get ready for your baby's arrival depends on the person you are and the birth you want: you may concentrate on your fitness, learn self-help techniques to give you the confidence to trust your body and the tools to help you cope, spend time writing a birth plan, choosing a birth partner (see Who will be at the birth?, page 133), or focusing on the practical things that make life easier around the birth.

There are no guarantees that if you prepare carefully the birth will be easy: you cannot hold yourself responsible for a baby in a poor position or a midwife unable to offer much practical support, for example. Circumstances can and should alter decisions, but planning and forethought usually make labour more manageable than it might otherwise have been.

A woman who is well-prepared can face the challenges knowing that most of the decisions she makes will be the right ones and that she will accept help gladly if it becomes necessary, regardless of her previous intentions.

Birth is not just about making babies. It is also about making strong, capable and confident mothers, able to make their own decisions and take on the responsibility for raising a child.

Body works

If you are fit and supple you are more likely to use your body well during labour and are therefore less likely to need intervention. If you have a Caesarean section, moving about afterwards will be easier and you will recover faster.

The basic elements of physical fitness are strength, suppleness and stamina. Strength and suppleness enable you to use positions which make labour easier and less painful; stamina helps you to keep going if your labour is long.

You can build stamina by taking a brisk walk or swimming regularly during pregnancy. If you do not normally take much exercise start gently, work up slowly and aim for at least three twenty-minute sessions a week. For any form of exercise it is sensible to warm up first and cool down afterwards; the golden rule is listen to your body. There is no sense in pushing yourself to exercise so hard that you feel exhausted afterwards.

Be cautious about activities which could raise your temperature or tempt you to push yourself too far, such as competitive sports or aerobics; and about taking up any new form of exercise unless the class is specially for pregnant women or your teacher knows that you are pregnant and is able to advise you. Talk to your doctor or midwife if you have any concerns about exercise.

Flexibility

Do these exercises every day to reduce stiffness and make your pelvic area more flexible. If you feel pain in your pubic joint stop doing them: your ligaments are already sufficiently stretchy.

- **Cat:** kneel on all fours, tilt your pelvis down as though you were tucking your tail under, then straighten your back. Rock your pelvis several times like this, then twist it from side to side, using your waist muscles. You can also do this exercise standing up, with your knees straight or slightly bent.
- **Tailor:** to help to relax the muscles of your inner thighs, sit on the floor with a straight back. Bring the soles of your feet together and your heels as close to your body as you can without straining. Stretch your knees apart and hold this for up to a few minutes.
- **Frog:** kneel and sit back on your heels; stretch your knees as wide apart as is comfortable. Relax your shoulders and make your back feel wider, then lift up from your waist and lean forward from the hip until your hands rest on the floor. Keeping your back straight, hold the position for up to a few minutes.

Using your body effectively saves energy, avoids strain and helps if you have an episiotomy, an assisted delivery or a Caesarean birth. When standing or walking, lengthen your spine, relax your neck muscles and imagine your head is balanced like a ping-pong ball on a water jet. When you have been sitting, use your arms to shift your weight to the edge of the chair. Keep your back straight, swing your body forward from the hips, think 'up' and rise smoothly without twisting your body or pushing off with your hands. The movement should feel light.

To get out of bed, roll on to your side, push up to a sitting position using your arms and swing your legs over the edge of the bed. Think 'up' and rise as you would from a chair. Practise until the movements become a habit.

Damage limitation

Your perineum is the tissue around the entrance to the vagina and it is designed to stretch and change shape as the baby's head presses on it during birth. The part between the vagina and anus is the most vulnerable, especially if a baby arrives very rapidly, or you are lying on your back so that gravity adds extra pressure. If you have an assisted delivery or the baby needs to be born right away with no opportunity for your perineum to stretch gently, it may be necessary to make an episiotomy, a small cut in this tissue.

Women generally have excellent powers of recovery after birth so the perineum usually heals quickly. It is not always possible to avoid an episiotomy or tear, but you can reduce the risk of damage:

- Prepare the tissue by massaging it daily after a shower or bath, from about thirty-four weeks. Work vitamin E or wheatgerm oil (or any pure vegetable oil) into the tissue for about five minutes, then stretch it gently with your thumbs, until you feel a burning sensation. Ask your partner to help if your bump gets in the way. After a week or two the tissue will feel much more yielding.
- During labour, avoid lying on your back to push. Even if you are propped up this adds the effects of gravity to the pressure on your perineum. Lying on your side, kneeling or standing with support avoids this extra pressure and there tends to be less sideways stretch on your perineum in these positions.
- Tell your midwife that an intact perineum (without an episiotomy or a tear) is important to you and ask her to help you. Listen if she asks you to stop pushing so that she can ease your baby's head out; pant like a dog on a hot day instead.

Mind matters

Some women find a normal labour nightmarish while others say with all honesty that a difficult labour was a positive experience. What makes the difference is the way you approach it. The end of pregnancy comes a day at a time so there is plenty of opportunity to develop a positive mindset.

When you imagine pain or not being able to cope with labour and feel panic rising you may notice anxiety symptoms such as a dry

---

Manage your thoughts

- Face your fears and accept that every experience has positive and negative aspects. Try not to magnify the negative or focus on what *might* happen.
- Take control, find out your options and decide what you prefer.
- Share responsibility for the way your birth goes instead of holding your doctor or midwife completely responsible or viewing every problem as your own fault.
- Ask for what you need, without taking a refusal personally. A single incident is not something that is likely to happen repeatedly.
- Set no rules about how you should or should not give birth, so that you cannot feel guilty if you break them, and you will not be upset if other people do.
- Use strategies to encourage yourself: write down the names of women you know who had the sort of birth you want and think 'if she can do it, so can I'; jot down what makes you feel you can handle the situation so that you can refer to it when your confidence wavers; stick affirmations (see Box below) on cupboard doors.
- Find the middle ground: birth is neither completely awful nor completely wonderful; nobody is either perfect or a failure.
- Concentrate on all the positive things about giving birth.

Affirmations

Affirmations are phrases that resonate with how you feel or would like to feel. Some women write out phrases which speak to them and they put them around the house where they will chance upon them during the weeks before the birth. Affirmations can help to change negative thought patterns. For example:

- I want to make my own choices. It is all right to be afraid of the responsibility.
- I can trust my inner feelings. I face my fears and learn courage.
- I can give birth. (Names of supporters) will help me.
- I know what to do for myself and my baby.
- I am perfectly designed to give birth. My body knows what to do.
- I accept that I am afraid, but I do not need to let fear control me.
- My baby and I are safe, no matter how I feel.
- People will listen when I ask for something.
- I will allow myself to receive love and support from other people.
- Pain is not a punishment.

mouth or butterflies in your stomach. These sensations are not caused by the birth; they are linked to your thoughts about what *might* happen. How you think affects how you feel.

To have the birth they want most women need to control how they think (see Manage your thoughts, page 125). Some women try to deal with fear by ignoring it. They read nothing and ask no questions; they concentrate their preparations for the baby on choosing nursery equipment rather than by going to antenatal classes. People learn very quickly to avoid uncomfortable feelings, but some fears just keep on surfacing until you face them.

Whatever sort of birth you want, accept the challenges that go with your choice. A long labour cannot be accelerated at home, for example, and a natural birth can be harder to achieve in some hospitals. Draw together all the resources you need to help you to feel confident in yourself, not entirely reliant on others.

Intuition and instinct

A woman giving birth taps into the primitive part of her brain which controls instinctive behaviour. She chooses positions intuitively, reaching out for help if she needs to move. She may cling to a helping hand or brush it away impatiently; she may be silent or rather noisy. When her contractions are strong she may seem unaware that anyone else is there, or she may lose confidence and need encouragement. There are many ways to cope with labour.

Instinctive behaviour is linked to the functioning of the right lobe of the brain, the part which influences creativity and imagination. Logical thought and intellectual reasoning are linked to the left brain. In response to stress the body releases the hormone cortisol, which helps to shift leadership from the left to the right lobe, short-cutting logical thought so that you act quickly and decisively. Cortisol is released during labour (see Birth hormones, page 34).

In a tricky driving situation, a back-seat driver issuing instructions is confusing because you become preoccupied with what they are telling you instead of acting instinctively. In the same way, a midwife who asks questions or performs intrusive examinations, or a birth partner who gives unnecessary instructions, prevents you from using your instinct during labour.

The left lobe of the brain distinguishes parts of wholes and the right lobe integrates parts into wholes; in other words, the left brain sees each tree while the right brain sees a whole forest. If you make rational decisions about what positions you should adopt, or stick to rules about how you should behave during labour, you see the individual trees, but lose your vision of the forest. Shifting control to the left brain overrides your intuitive knowledge of how to help yourself.

Instinct and intuition are closely linked, and continuity of care makes it easier to use these sources of knowledge (see Women's ways of knowing, page 21). It is not necessary to be emotionally close to someone to tune into their wavelength, but you need to build a relationship to use intuition. A midwife who knows you, for example, has less need to stick rigidly to a textbook or protocol.

If you are well-prepared for labour, you will know instinctively what to do at the time and can trust your instincts. Birthing skills help you to have the birth you want by providing a background, not a set of rules.

Developing intuition

There is no need to search for true intuition. Given the right circumstances and a prepared mind, it just comes. The more that external knowledge confirms your intuition the easier it is to trust the sign or the feeling that accompanies it.

- You need to feel safe. You cannot use instinct if somebody is breathing down your neck and judging your performance, or if you feel unable to express yourself in a responsible way.
- You need to be confident about your preparations, cultivate a stillness or readiness (to shift control to the right brain), and believe that you will know what to do at the time.
- You have to be willing to allow it to happen, like a baby bird who launches itself from the nest and trusts it knows how to fly.

Birthing skills

Your birth experience will always be more manageable if you feel relaxed and confident. Coping strategies reduce tension, prevent panic and help you to be less dependent on drugs – during labour or post-operatively. You can learn some of these skills at classes (see Choosing antenatal classes, page 132).

Pain-relieving techniques include the sorts of things you might use in daily life: applying heat or massage to an area that aches in order to block the nerve fibres that transmit pain messages to your brain, for example, or focusing on something else to bombard the nerve fibres with competing messages. Such techniques have no side effects and can be used singly or in combination. To keep the relief going, move from one technique to another when the effect wears off.

You cannot know in advance exactly what skills you will need, so aim to acquire those that you *might* need and practice until you feel they become part of you. They are tools to help you give birth as comfortably as possible and some of them may turn out to be indispensable.

Relaxation

Tension makes pain less tolerable and it affects your breathing. If you start to panic, your body stiffens, your breathing speeds up, and you may over-breathe or hyperventilate. This makes you feel light-headed and out of control, a frightening sensation that can create more panic.

You can avoid getting into this state by relaxing into pain instead of fighting it. Your uterus will work more effectively and your body will release endorphins and enkephalins, the hormones that help to relieve pain naturally. When you are tense these are inhibited by stress hormones.

A calm and confident approach to labour can help you to relax and one of the keys to staying relaxed is to be able to detect tension and release it consciously. Most women have a weak spot, often their hands, shoulders or jaw, where tension shows up over and over again, so they concentrate on keeping this spot relaxed.

During labour you may need to check your face, shoulders and hands at the start and finish of every contraction, so that tension does not get a chance to build up unnoticed. Practise these movements and keep checking through the day until you can recognise the smallest degree of tension and let it go:

- Pull your shoulders down, then release them.
- Clench your fists, then loosen your fingers.
- Tense your jaw, then let your whole face relax.

Breathing

Breathing and relaxation go hand in hand: change the one and you change the other. Relax completely and you will notice that your breathing is gentle and quiet and effortless.

The strength of labour contractions can 'take your breath away', a sensation which makes your body stiffen involuntarily. When your breathing becomes fast and jerky, your face, hands or shoulders are likely to be tense, which can quickly develop into panic. You can avoid this by deliberately calming your breathing.

Practise slowing your breathing slightly, emphasising the 'out' breath. When this is comfortable lengthen the 'out' breath slightly and notice your stomach gently rise and fall. There is no need to rush: when you have exhaled fully there will be a momentary pause and your lungs will inflate effortlessly. Look for another slight pause when you have breathed in fully, but without holding your breath.

During labour, sigh out fully at the start and finish of each contraction. Check your face, hands and shoulders, letting go any tension. Keep your breathing slow and quiet, concentrating on the 'out' breath and the slight pause.

Focusing

At a party, most people do not notice a headache which might trouble them at work; concentrating fully on something else takes one's mind off discomfort. This strategy can be surprisingly effective during labour. Experiment until you find visual images that feel relaxing. The last three of the following examples may help when pain is severe and you need to focus on something simple or mechanical:

- Think of a surge of energy bathed in white light; or a powerful wave that you ride on a surfboard until it reaches the beach; or, as each contraction begins, imagine diving into a deep, cool pool and rising gently to the surface as it fades.
- Imagine a red beach ball containing your pain. Feel the pain evaporate as you watch it deflate slowly.
- You are lying on a beach in warm sunshine. Waves wash over you and recede, taking tension with them. Some of them make your body float briefly before setting you down and flowing gently away.
- Think of a flower opening, petal by petal, a dove circling overhead and flying away, or a pebble making circular ripples when dropped into a still pool.
- Fix your attention on a clock, slowly counting with each tick of the second hand; count the tiles on a roof, the slats on a Venetian blind, or the repeat pattern on curtains or a bed cover.
- Concentrate on a picture or object (a candle flame works well if you are at home) during each contraction. Carefully observe the shapes and colours.
- Using earphones, turn up the volume on a personal stereo so that the sound fills your mind during contractions.

Touch and temperature

Most people have used massage to soothe an ache at some time or other, or a hot water bottle or an ice pack to relieve pain. In early labour massage can take your mind off contractions and help you to unwind. Ask your partner to try different types on your face, shoulders or feet until you discover what helps you to relax. Try a wooden back massager; or slip two tennis balls into a sock and roll it up and down your back.

Stroking round under your bump with light pressure from a relaxed hand can release surface tension and soothe an ache. Later on, firm pressure on your lower back will help to relieve backache.

A hot or cold compress can relieve pain by changing the temperature. Wrap a hot-water bottle or an ice pack in a towel before applying it. Your body will get used to the new sensation after a while and pain messages will leak through again, so alternate temperature changes with massage to keep up the relief.

Choosing antenatal classes

Antenatal classes differ in size, approach and the subjects covered. Some are discussion-based and focus on practical birthing skills and caring for a new baby; others are more formal, with lectures on different topics given by a midwife, a health visitor or a physiotherapist. In some classes, you learn about your choices and how to help yourself; in others, you are told what is expected of you in hospital.

Classes run by midwives employed by your local health authority are free. The National Childbirth Trust and the Active Birth Centre make a charge, but they are more likely to teach self-help techniques such as massage and birth positions.

Your midwife may give you details of all the classes in your area, or you may find private classes advertised on the hospital notice board. Many women find the right class for their needs by asking friends or neighbours for a recommendation.

- You may meet women who live nearby at a class run by your local midwife; and women on the same wavelength at classes further afield which has been recommended by a friend. If you hope to get to know other pregnant women and develop friendships, ask the teacher how often her groups stay in touch with each other.
- A small group may suit you best if you want to ask questions and discuss birth, but if you prefer to merge into a crowd look for a large, lecture-based class.
- If you have a disability, make sure the class can accommodate your needs.
- If you are on your own, you may prefer a women-only group; but your mum or a friend can usually accompany you to a course for couples.
- Small classes get booked up early; think ahead if you would prefer a small group.
- Try to find a class which involves men as equals if your husband or partner is keen to be involved. Some classes treat men as onlookers.
- If you want a natural birth, ask whether self-help and alternative approaches will be covered. Some classes assume that everyone will have an epidural.

Who will be at the birth?

A good birth partner is a willing slave who does whatever makes you more comfortable. Anyone can be at a home birth, including grandparents, children or the family pet; and you can potter about to keep yourself occupied or take your mind off contractions. In hospital, there may be little diversion other than pacing your room or the corridors, so the right companion can make all the difference.

If your partner is keen to be there, try to attend antenatal classes where he can learn what to expect and what he can do to help you. Concern and tenderness are more important than first-class massage skills, but sensitive support given at the right moment can raise your pain threshold and help you to cope. Some women find dealing with contractions a lonely experience without a companion; many want plenty of encouragement, but even if your birth partner just stays by your side you will value his or her presence.

Forty years ago, a father had a hard time if he wanted to see his child born. Today, he has an equally hard time escaping; but birth is not a spectator sport and the role of birth partner does not suit all men. Some men worry that they will not be able to help and some women are afraid that their partner will be traumatised by what he sees and might look at them differently afterwards. Some women are afraid that their partner will take over and tell them what to do; and, while they try to follow instructions, they will lose their instinct and end up confused.

Whether having your partner present at the birth is right for you as a couple may depend on the nature of your relationship. Not wanting to be together at the birth is no reflection on the strength of your relationship or your partner's fitness for fatherhood.

A birth partner needs to be a supportive companion and advocate. A friend or relative could be your companion, and more than one birth partner can be a great help if one of you is ambivalent or if the labour is long and gruelling.

If you have no close relatives or friends living nearby to help out around the birth you could consider engaging a doula (see the Baby Directory website listed in the Directory). The title comes from the ancient Greek word for a servant or handmaiden and today they provide companionship, support and practical assistance to mothers around the time of birth. They are trained to act as a birth partner if you wish.

Children at the birth

There is rarely any opposition to having children around at a home birth and it may be possible to have an older child present in a small maternity unit. Talk to your midwife as early as possible, however; she may need to get used to the idea and you will want the child to feel welcome.

Unless children are old enough to be left unsupervised, arrange for someone other than your birth partner to be there to look after them. If you go into labour at night they may be asleep and during the day there is not much to interest them, so they will not want to watch contractions for long.

Toddlers tend to take birth in their stride provided you are calm, but they get upset when you cannot talk to them during contractions. Children who are old enough to understand about birth need careful preparation and someone there to explain things and to reassure them. They need to know that you may be bad-tempered or make a noise and that it may not be possible for them to be present if there is a problem. School-age children often worry about practical things, such as who will make their tea or find their gym kit for school; but some of them enjoy spending part of the time making a cake to celebrate the baby's arrival.

Teenagers tend to feel responsible and protective towards you. They need the reassurance of knowing that you are not depending on them and that they can stay or go, depending on what feels right to them at the time.

Being present when a brother or sister is born can be a very special experience for a child, but the older they are the more impact it can have. Plan as carefully as possible to make their first experience of birth a positive one.

Birth plans

A birth plan sets down your preferences to help staff you may not have seen before to help you. If you know the midwife who will deliver your baby you can discuss the birth with her; if not, write anything that is important to you in a letter and have it attached to your notes or give it to the staff when you go into hospital.

Several closely spaced pages of instructions may not be read, so indicate the approach you prefer and any points that are especially important to you (see Birth options, page 136). Word the letter carefully – if you put in writing that you do not want an epidural you will not get one, even if you change your mind!

You may want to discuss your options and the implications with your midwife before deciding what to write on your birth plan. When you think seriously about birth and your choices you often become more realistic and more flexible.

Birth options

- Would you want a slow labour speeded up? Would you prefer to be monitored by a belt or a scalp electrode? (See Quick Guide: Assistance in labour, page 96).
- What pain relief do you prefer? (See Quick Guide: Other methods of pain relief, pages 72–3).
- Would you like to eat or drink when you feel like it? To have encouragement and practical ideas to help you to avoid drugs?
- Do you want an 'active' birth, moving freely and choosing your own positions?
- Do you want to push in an upright position, deliver your baby standing or lying on your side, or be helped to avoid an episiotomy or tear?
- Is it important to you to avoid routine internal examinations?
- Would you like more than one birth partner, or members of your family to be present when, or soon after, your baby arrives?
- Is it important to you that people use your name rather than 'my dear', or that they respect your privacy and knock before they come into the room?
- Does a 'gentle' birth – a calm atmosphere, low lights and no unnecessary chatter when your baby is born – appeal to you?
- Would you like your baby given to you straight away or cleaned and wrapped up first? Do you want to be told your baby's sex or discover it for yourself?
- How do you want the cord to be cut and the placenta delivered?

- Do you mind if students are present during labour? If your birth is unusual, how do you feel about an audience? Do you want only essential staff there?
- If you have a general anaesthetic for a Caesarean birth, would you like someone to take photos and record your baby's first cries if possible, or to describe the birth to you afterwards? Do you want to breastfeed as soon as you can?
- Would you like someone to chat to you during a Caesarean under epidural, or to have a personal stereo with your choice of music? Do you want the screen lowered so that you can see your baby being born?

All set and ready to go

In the last month or so, most women get an urge to have everything ready for when contractions start in earnest. When the final preparations are complete you can let go, knowing that you have done your best to ensure you have the birth you want.

Midwifery unit or hospital

If you are having your baby away from home, you may want to pack your bag about four weeks before your baby is due, in case the birth is early. You will be given a list of things to take in, such as toiletries, sanitary towels, baby clothes and nappies.

Even if you are planning a home birth, make sure that you have enough petrol for the journey to hospital and that your birth partner knows where to go, including the door to use at night and the parking arrangements.

Home birth

Your midwife will bring everything she needs, including gas and air, and will discuss anything she would like you to provide: for example, a flat surface for her equipment, a strong torch or a fan heater. If you think you might need pethidine, get a prescription from your GP and keep the drug in your fridge until required.

There is surprisingly little mess or disruption at a home birth, but you may like to protect your mattress or carpet with plastic sheeting from a DIY store or builder's merchant, especially for a water birth.

You could prepare bulbs, flowers or autumn leaves to brighten the bathroom or birth room, or line up tea lights in saucers on a shelf to light at intervals during labour. Some people like to use essential oils in a room burner, but some midwives find them overpowering. You may want to collect things for your comfort (see Useful items for labour, page 140) and plan snacks to sustain your birth partner and midwife. Special treats to eat contribute to a happy atmosphere.

Water birth

If you are having a water birth at home, or want to be certain that you can have one in hospital, you will need to hire a pool (see Arranging a water birth, page 91). At home, site it where the floor is strong (a stone or concrete floor is ideal). If the birth is to take place upstairs, put it close to or preferably over a load-bearing wall. Some people place lengths of scaffolding board or thick plywood across the joists to help spread the weight.

There is usually plenty of time to assemble a pool in early labour; they slot together easily, even if you are not normally gifted at DIY. In hospital, they take about twenty minutes to fill. At home, it depends on the time needed for the water to heat. Turn the immersion heater to high and cover the pool between fillings.

If the pool has a soft liner, you may want to put an old duvet down to pad the floor underneath and some women mould a beanbag into shape to lean on before filling the pool. A plastic stool can be useful to get in and out of the water, or to sit on in the pool; and a birth ball (see Active Birth Centre in the Directory) makes convenient seating for your partner or midwife.

Useful items for labour

Wherever you give birth you will find it easier to cope if you are not too hot or cold and you have things to eat and to pass the time.

- **General comfort:** v-shaped back pillow; beanbag; inflatable 65 cm. birth ball to sit or lean on (more supportive than a bean bag); personal stereo; music/story tapes or CDs; games, books, other pastimes; camera and film, video recorder; hot-water bottle to make a hot or cold compress; bucket (pad the rim with a thick towel) to sit on if pressure underneath is uncomfortable; a picture or flowers to focus on; aromatherapy oils; socks for cold feet.
- **Refreshments:** cans of juice in a six-pack cool-bag (to drink or to apply counter-pressure for backache); ice cubes to chill drinks or make an ice pack; biscuits, stewed fruit or yogurt for energy; mineral or fruit-flavoured water; herbal tea bags; special treats, snacks, sandwiches for your birth partner.
- **For a dry mouth:** sips of water; small natural sponge to moisten lips; lip balm; fruit-flavoured ice chips, lollies or ice-pops (insulate in kitchen foil to travel).
- **To stay cool:** loose t-shirt, cotton shirt or nightie (a change is refreshing); battery or pleated paper fan; mineral water or water-filled plant spray; face fresheners.
- **For backache:** talc or oil for massage; hot-water bottle for a hot or cold compress; frozen sports gel pack; wooden back massager.
- **For a water birth:** bath sheet or towelling robe; dry t-shirts, bras or crop tops to wear in the pool if you want; rubber ring or foam pillow covered with polythene for support; swimming trunks for your partner if he wants to get in the pool; small sieve to remove debris if necessary.

Countdown

You may like to plan ahead to make life easier for two or three months around the birth. The last few weeks of pregnancy can be tiring, so never stand when you can sit or sit when you could lie down; and never refuse an offer of help.

32–34 weeks

- Cut down on shopping by bulk buying items like detergent or pet food.
- Fill your freezer and store cupboard with the basics for simple meals; stock up with biscuits for visitors and things like soap if relatives will be staying.
- Check arrangements for hiring a birth pool or TENS machine; or engaging a doula or maternity nurse.
- Start perineal massage using vitamin E or wheatgerm oil (see page 124).
- Wherever you plan to give birth, check that your partner knows where to park at the hospital and what door to use at night, to reduce the pressure on him.

34–36 weeks

- For a first baby, start using basic positions (see Quick Guides: Complementary therapies to turn a baby and Help your baby into a good position, pages 48 and 49–50).
- If your baby is lying in an awkward position, discuss external cephalic version (see page 118) with your consultant.
- Have a rest after lunch and practise breathing and relaxation skills every day.
- Protect your mattress with a plastic sheet or an old shower curtain in case your waters break in bed.
- Make arrangements for the care of your other children around the birth.

- Buy stamps, birth announcement cards and thank-you notes to acknowledge gifts as they arrive.
- If you are having a Caesarean make sure you have plenty of help afterwards.

36–38 weeks

- Restock your freezer and store cupboard if you have used some of the items.
- Check that you have batteries for a cassette recorder and film for your camera.
- Collect together what you need for comfort at the birth. Pack your hospital bag.
- If it is your second or later baby, start using the basic positions.
- If you have a child staying with someone else while you are in hospital, pack a bag for him. Write a diary of your toddler's day to help whoever looks after him.
- After a Caesarean section you may run out of energy more quickly than you expected. Put sleeping and nappy-changing equipment for the baby upstairs and downstairs to save climbing stairs.

38–40 weeks

- Get new videos and story tapes from the library to entertain your toddler for an hour or so every day, while you put your feet up.
- Arrange for someone to feed your pets while you're in labour.
- Record a message on your answering machine giving news of the birth. Ask people to visit after 3 p.m. to avoid visitors arriving at all hours.
- Plan some outings for after your due date so that you have something to look forward to if you go overdue.
- Make a note of everyone who offers help: you can ask five people for help once or twice but you may not like to ask one person ten times.
- Other things to remember . . . .

In brief

- Nothing can guarantee that the birth will turn out the way you want, but good preparation makes most situations more manageable.
- If you are fit and supple you will be able to use your body well during birth; you will also recover more rapidly, especially after a Caesarean birth.
- How you think affects how you feel. Most women need to adopt a positive frame of mind in order to have the birth they want.
- Birthing skills provide a background for handling labour, not a set of rules.
- When you are well prepared you are more likely to feel confident and relaxed, so that you know intuitively what to do at the time.
- Writing a birth plan involves thinking about your options and your individual needs so it can make you more realistic and flexible.

Quick Guide: For birth partners

Discuss what the mother prefers beforehand so that she can trust you to make the final decision. Be there for her. Stay supportive, even if she gets cross!

- In early labour, aim to make time pass and keep morale up. Create a relaxed and cheerful atmosphere, even if anxious.
- Take your lead from her, offering help or standing back as seems best. Accept and understand if she rejects your efforts.
- Act as her spokesperson for the staff, but be sensitive if she changes her mind about something.
- Stay quiet during contractions. Chattering drags her into conscious, rational thought as she tries to listen or respond.
- Remind her that she knows what to do for herself and her baby; reassure her that you will be there and that although she feels afraid she is safe.
- Give feedback about what she does that seems to work. This is more helpful than sympathy.
- Remind her to breathe gently, emphasising the 'out' breath, and to relax her hands, shoulders and jaw. Gently stroke her hair or palm, massage her back or feet, unless she indicates that she can't bear to be touched.
- Give her something to focus on through strong contractions: count slowly or quietly or describe a place you both like.
- Put your arms round her or let her lean on you, adjusting your position when the contraction is over. If you are supporting her weight, protect your back: keep it straight, bend your knees slightly and use your thigh muscles.
- If she wanted a natural birth but intervention becomes essential, praise and comfort her afterwards. Even after a straightforward birth women need reassurance that they coped well.

1

2

3

4

5

6

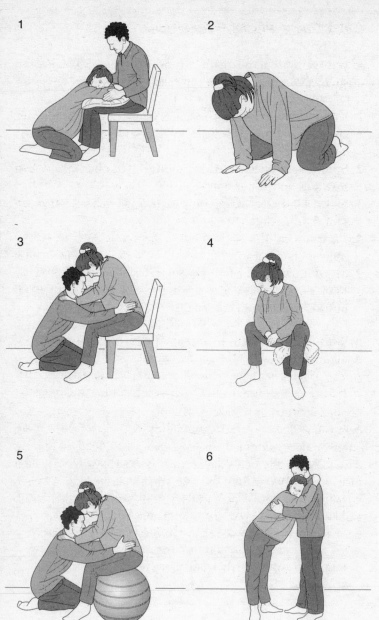

Quick Guide: Positions for labour

If you want an active birth, try out these positions during pregnancy to see which you can relax in:

1. Kneel on something soft, such as a pillow, with your knees apart. Lean on to a bed, a chair, a bean bag, a birth ball or your partner.
2. Spread your knees to make room for your bump and lean forwards on to your hands.
3. Sit on a low stool facing your partner; stretch your arms up round his neck.
4. Pad the rim of a bucket with a towel; sit on it to relieve pressure underneath.
5. Sit on a birth ball and rock your pelvis or bounce gently.
6. Walk slowly, leaning on your partner, a wall or a handy piece of furniture when a contraction starts.

In any position, rock or rotate your pelvis or move your body slowly and rhythmically from side to side, back and forth or in an oval shape.

If you end up on the bed on your back with your knees flopped apart after an internal examination, your partner can help you to change position as follows: with your feet on their outer borders, slide one foot towards your bottom, lowering that knee to the bed. Using your hands for support, lean forward until your body is over your knee, then roll into a kneeling position. When you are on both knees facing the side of the bed you can put your arms around your partner's neck for support or move round to lean on the bedhead.

Quick Guide: Positions for birth

Upright positions enlist the help of gravity and even out pressure to help avoid a tear. When your baby's head crowns, you may instinctively move into a horizontal position. Experiment with your birth partner to find practical positions.

1. Squat between your partner's legs while he (or she) sits on a chair; lean into his lap with your arms over his knees for support.
2. Squat on the bed with your partner and a midwife standing either side with one arm round your back to support you. Put your arms round their necks.
3. Semi-squat with support as above, but on a mattress or sheet on the floor.
4. Kneel and lean on to your partner, the bedhead or a pile of pillows.
5. Stand, leaning against your partner with his arms supporting you under the armpits and his hands clasping yours to ease underarm pressure.
6. Lie on your side: your partner supports your upper leg during a contraction.

If you have an epidural you may be able to roll on to your side, with help.

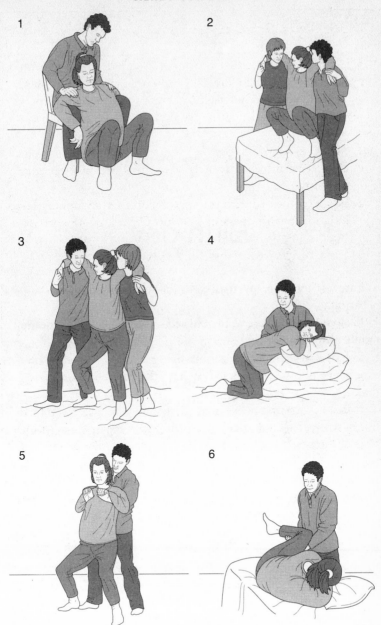

7

Birth day

Whatever your perspective, your baby's birth day is a special occasion.

Is labour a challenge to be relished or an ordeal to be endured, a purely physical experience or one with a spiritual element? You may feel that a healthy baby is a satisfying enough outcome for any experience of birth, or you may believe that there is more to it than that.

If this is your first baby, or the first time you have given birth in this way, treat labour with optimism and respect; expect to learn from the experience. You do not have to please other people or take the conventional route. Having the birth you want is not about performing the 'right' way, nor does it follow that once you have made the initial decisions things will turn out the way you expect.

People who do things perfectly have usually had plenty of practice. If you set your sights impossibly high the experience may not live up to your expectations, and if you do not think you deserve a good birth, you may sabotage your chances when the time comes. Believe in yourself in order to help other people to believe in you.

Like making love, giving birth is possible more or less anywhere, but definitely easier in some situations than others. Contractions are controlled by the same delicate hormones that are responsible for orgasm and they are just as easily inhibited by disturbance or anxiety. Endorphins, the body's natural opiates, can only relieve pain if you are sufficiently relaxed for them to flow well.

Labour will be easier if you are in a place where you feel secure and you can labour in the way which feels right for you, with the support of a partner and a midwife you know and trust. If something doesn't work, relax, and find another way, one which works better.

You are more likely to have the birth you want if you are well-prepared, trust your instinct and make individual choices based on self-knowledge; but however it turns out, this is the birth of your child. Welcome the experience.

Birth patterns

Labour consists of an overture and three movements, or linked stages. Before it begins, the cervix or neck of the uterus, which is tightly closed during pregnancy, thins out until it forms part of the main body of the uterus. Contractions may stop and start for several days or build up gradually over a number of hours.

In the first stage of labour, your uterus contracts more and more strongly to dilate your cervix for the baby to pass through. To some extent this is influenced by body type: you might be a natural sprinter, able to produce great power and energy in short bursts, or you may have the stamina more suited to running a marathon.

Once labour starts, a speedy uterus gets the job over in a few hours, although the contractions can be so relentless that you feel swept along like a tiny boat in a raging torrent, longing to be set down on the shore. If your uterus is built for stamina, contractions tend to be much gentler, but they sometimes go on and on long after you have lost interest. This sort of labour can be fun at first and exciting at the finish but it is tough when exhaustion sets in; it makes similar physical and emotional demands to running a marathon.

When your cervix is fully dilated, the second stage of labour begins: pushing your baby through the birth canal to be born. For some women, this is hard work; for others, it is painless and satisfying: they feel their body does most of the work. The third stage, the delivery of the placenta or afterbirth, completes the birth.

The progress of labour is affected by body type, but also by the position of your baby and whether you are tense or relaxed. If your baby is lying awkwardly, labour may take longer as the contractions turn him into a better position; if you are anxious or stressed for some reason, it may take longer for your hormones to settle down and stop inhibiting effective contractions.

The best way of making labour easier is to stay as relaxed as possible so that your uterus can work with its maximum efficiency to birth your baby.

Going overdue

Plan activities for after your due date, so that you have something to look forward to instead of sitting around waiting for contractions.

Some women use traditional methods of starting labour off, but these only tend to work if their cervix is ripe and ready for labour. You may want to consult a qualified practitioner for individual advice when using complementary therapies.

Things you can try

- Go for a long walk, eat a hot curry or other spicy food, try nipple stimulation (ten to fifteen minutes, several times a day), or lovemaking.
- If you are slightly dilated, ask your midwife to 'sweep' your membranes (separate them from the wall of the uterus). This increases prostaglandin production although it may be uncomfortable at the time. The mucus plug may come away or you may have colicky pains afterwards.
- A homoeopath might suggest Caulophyllum or Pulsatilla to help ripen your cervix.
- Acupuncture treatment over a few days can help to ripen the

cervix. A pin may be left in place so that you can stimulate the point between treatments.

- Aromatherapists may recommend clary sage for massage or in a bath.
- A clinic in Malta claims a dose of 50 ml. of castor oil mixed with a tablespoon of sugar and the juice of six squeezed oranges usually succeeds if the cervix is ripe.
- A medical herbalist might suggest capsules of Evening Primrose oil, or a tincture based on Blue Cohosh, to initiate labour.

Ready, steady, go!

In the last few weeks of pregnancy you may get Braxton Hicks contractions that tone the muscles of your uterus ready for labour. They feel like gentle tightenings, or from time to time your abdomen feels hard and round like a football. They often come and go in waves for several days and may build up so that you are convinced labour has begun, only to disappear when you decide to do something about it.

Before labour starts, some women get some diarrhoea and others get a strong 'nesting urge', a strange unsettled feeling or even an urge to paint the bathroom or clean the oven! You may notice Braxton Hicks contractions come more frequently and last twenty to thirty seconds each (see Contractions, page 152).

A few hours or several days before labour starts, you might have a 'show': the mucus plug that seals the cervix comes away, looking like a small blob of blood-streaked jelly. There is no need to do anything about this, although tell your midwife if there is fresh bleeding.

The waters break for 10–15 per cent of women in public. It rarely happens, if it does the baby's head usually acts as a cork, preventing most of the fluid from escaping. Provided the fluid is clear or straw-coloured, there is no great drama. Just contact your midwife or the hospital to let them know, although you may not feel contractions for several hours. You are unlikely to dilate so fast that you do not get to hospital in time, especially with your first baby.

The most common way for labour to start is with regular, increasingly strong contractions that come anything from twenty minutes to five minutes apart. They are more distinct than Braxton Hicks contractions, but neither painful nor dramatic at first. When you feel you need support, ask your midwife to come and check you, or phone the hospital for advice (see Quick Guide: Is it labour? page 170).

Going to hospital can disturb the hormones that control contractions, so they may fade away temporarily, resuming when you are at ease again. Feeling upset or pressured can also switch off labour; if you feel uncomfortable with your midwife, tactfully ask the sister-in-charge if someone else may care for you.

In hospital, you usually have a single room for labour and birth. Your midwife takes your blood pressure and temperature, feels your abdomen, and examines you internally to see how far dilated you are. She may suggest monitoring your baby's heartbeat for twenty minutes to get a base reading (this is optional), then you and your partner will be left to your own devices.

If you wish, you could stay fully dressed and walk around to pass the time, having a short rest period every hour. You will be shown the bell to press if you need help.

During labour, your midwife is likely to examine you internally approximately every four hours and keep an eye on you in between. She will check your baby's position and heartbeat, take your blood pressure and provide pain relief if needed. When you are ready to push, a second midwife usually arrives to help.

For a home birth, your midwife will check you in early labour and you can carry on as usual, breathing through contractions when you need to. She may go off to make other calls but she will stay once you are in established labour, making sure that you and the baby are all right and helping you to cope.

Contractions

Braxton Hicks contractions last twenty to thirty seconds from start to finish and may be irregular. They often become stronger for a while and then fade away when you change position or are about to take them seriously. You can usually chat or distract yourself in between them. They may feel like tightenings in your abdomen; waves of period-like cramp, low down around your cervix; an ache that starts in your back and radiates round to the front; persistent, dull backache; cramp in your thighs or groin; being squeezed by a lycra belt which is too tight; or surges of energy that take your breath away.

Labour contractions come at regular five- to ten-minute intervals and last forty-five to fifty seconds. As labour progresses, they become longer, stronger and more frequent – every two to five minutes, and lasting sixty to ninety seconds. It can be hard to tell when your cervix starts to dilate, but at some point the contractions will feel more painful and purposeful.

At first, you have to stop what you are doing to relax and let them pass, but you need to concentrate on relaxing only when you have a contraction. As they strengthen and get closer together, you may have to consciously relax both during and between them. You may feel a sensation of breathlessness; strong, painful cramp-like sensations; persistent backache, peaking but never fading completely; or an instinct that you need help or reassurance.

Pushing contractions have a downward movement to them and when you experience them for the first time they often feel strangely familiar. Many women describe them as satisfying, but some find them painful. You may feel a catch, or make an involuntary sound in your throat; your knees may wobble if you are standing; or pressure from the baby's head may make you feel like opening your bowels.

Natural birth

Your individual experience of labour will depend on things such as the position of your baby, your emotional state and your body's physical attributes.

Thinning

In a first birth, this phase often forms part of a continuous sequence of contractions which eventually strengthen enough to dilate the cervix; but in later births, the cervix may thin out and dilate a couple of centimetres over the last week or two of pregnancy. You may be too excited or nervous to concentrate on anything for long, so have activities saved up to pass the time and take your mind off contractions (see Tips for natural birth, pages 155–6).

Early labour

As your cervix begins to dilate, the contractions settle down and become regular. You may need to relax consciously, greet each one with a slow breath out and breathe gently through it. This phase can go on for many hours, so pace yourself from the start and try not to take it too seriously too soon.

Strong labour

As labour progresses, your muscles work harder to dilate the cervix. When contractions last forty-five to fifty seconds, there will be little doubt in your mind that they mean business. You may need to concentrate so hard on staying relaxed that you cannot chat in between them. Just switch off and let instinct take over. Try to welcome each contraction, without feeling sorry for yourself.

No position will be comfortable, but leaning forwards, lying on your side, rocking your pelvis, moving your body in slow circles or getting in a deep warm bath or a birth pool, may help. The intense contractions that dilate the last rim of the cervix can be the most frustrating part of labour and you may feel overwhelmed, irritable or tearful.

Birth

When you are ready to push, the contractions change. Your midwife may ask you to hold back for a few contractions if you are not fully dilated; or there may be a short lull before your baby moves down the birth canal, stretches your pelvic floor and triggers the pushing reflex. Pushing takes from a few minutes to several hours as the baby turns to fit more easily through your pelvis. To push, you use some of the muscles used to pee. You may feel your throat close with a grunting sound, or the strong urge to bear down may feel like opening your bowels.

Afterwards

The placenta or afterbirth separates from the wall of the uterus and contractions seal the blood vessels naturally. Your baby's cord will continue to pulsate for several minutes, giving him extra blood and a gentler transition to breathing air. It can take an hour or so for the placenta to arrive, feeling soft and rather like a blancmange, but you could also have an injection to bring it away quickly. You can usually cuddle your baby immediately. Many women feel full of joy, although some feel rather bemused and disorientated.

Tips for natural birth

Try not to take the contractions too seriously too soon; plan tasks or activities that will help you to stay relaxed:

- Clean out a cupboard; write letters, send e-mails, address birth announcement cards; bake a cake, make meals to freeze; look through family photos, plan a holiday; watch a video, listen to music or story tapes; phone a friend to chat, or invite her for coffee; start a tapestry kit, a jigsaw, novel or magazine; play cards, scrabble, dominoes; go for a walk.
- At night, walk under the stars with your partner; take two paracetamol to reduce discomfort; have a candle-lit bath, a cup of cocoa, and try to sleep.
- Ask your midwife if she could visit you at home in early

---

labour, to reassure you and your partner that everything is going well.

- When the contractions demand attention, massage your abdomen with a relaxed hand, have a warm bath, cuddle a hot-water bottle, rock your body rhythmically.
- Move around and find comfortable positions that help you to relax.
- Keep the lights low if labour starts in the evening or at night – darkness tends to favour instinct over rational behaviour. When you are relaxed or your brain is at rest, your hormones flow more readily.
- Your contractions may be stronger in certain positions. If they are intense, rest for half an hour in a position that eases them, then get them going again.
- Wait until the contractions are as strong as you can bear (usually after 5 cm.) before entering a birth pool. Water can sap your energy if you stay in it for hours.
- A deep bath can ease pain – put towels down and block the overflow with Blu-Tack; or stand in a shower, directing the water onto your back or under your bump.
- Submit to pain rather than trying to control it; accept it instead of fighting it.
- Trust your body and your helpers. Consciously open up and let go.

Alternative therapies

Some of these alternative remedies are not suitable for use in pregnancy, but they can be used in labour to help reduce tension, regulate your contractions, relieve pain or reduce bleeding. A qualified therapist can give you individual advice; some will make up a birth kit or give advice by phone during labour.

Aromatherapy

Chamomile, geranium or lavender essential oils can help you relax and breathe calmly. Clary sage tones the muscles of the uterus and strengthens contractions. Bergamot or mandarin give you energy. Neroli, rose or jasmine reduce anxiety and boost confidence.

Some therapists suggest massaging your abdomen once or twice during labour with rose or geranium oil, individually or blended together. Try five drops of essential oil in a room burner, one drop in a teaspoonful of vegetable oil for massage, or four drops in a warm bath.

Herbalism

Motherwort or skullcap can relieve pain or distress and help you relax. Beth root and blue or black cohosh improve weak or irregular contractions. Raspberry leaf helps to regulate over-strong contractions. Ginseng gives energy. Drink teas throughout labour, make ice cubes to suck or make an infusion to use in compresses.

Homoeopathy

Caulophyllum can help to tone your uterus if you have previously had a slow labour. When pain is severe, try Aconite if you're anxious; Chamomile if you're impatient for labour to finish; Cimicifuga if pain moves from side to side and your belly feels tender, Gelsemium or Kali carb if pain is in your back and you feel weak. Arnica can help to avoid excessive bruising.

Acupuncture

During labour, this can encourage the release of endorphins, your body's natural pain-relieving chemicals. Some acupuncturists attend your labour and use needles on points on your ear, leg or foot; alternatively, you may be given a device like a TENS machine with electrodes to attach with sticky pads to certain points on your leg. After about twenty minutes of treatment you may begin to feel relaxed and sleepy.

Birth with technology

Technology can be a great help when a labour is not progressing, the mother or baby are becoming distressed, or there is reason to be concerned about their welfare.

Induction

Some doctors routinely suggest inducing labour when you are a week or two overdue. You may want to ask why it is necessary in your case and whether you could be monitored daily instead.

Statistically, the more overdue you go the greater the chance of foetal distress, leading to an emergency Caesarean section; but factors such as the length of your cycle are also important.

A prostaglandin pessary or gel is inserted to soften and thin your cervix. More than one dose can be given, but when you are overdue, a small dose may be enough. If your cervix has dilated a little, your waters may be broken, or a hormone drip set up and increased gradually to stimulate stronger contractions. Your baby should be monitored throughout (see Quick Guide: Assistance in labour, page 96).

Get into a comfortable position before drips and monitors are set up. You do not have to lie in bed, but if you change position, your baby may move and a belt monitor may need to be repositioned. An induced labour may be more painful, depending on things such as the baby's position and whether your uterus is ready for birth. If induction is essential, this is unavoidable; ask for pain relief if you need it.

Acceleration

If your contractions slow down during labour, a hormone drip could avoid a very long labour and possibly a Caesarean section. Make sure that labour really is established with strong, regular contractions, however; some women stop and start, or plod along gently for many hours until they are a few centimetres dilated, then their contractions strengthen naturally and they make good progress.

Technology tips

- Ask for gas and air if having a pessary inserted or your waters broken is painful. It can also help if the gel or pessaries give you colicky pains, which can be more uncomfortable than the true contractions that follow.
- Drips and belt monitors restrict your freedom to move so get comfortable on a beanbag or chair before they are set in place. You could change position from time to time and ask the midwife to reposition the monitors.
- Keep an open mind about having pethidine or an epidural. Intervention can make labour more painful and continuous monitoring can prevent you from moving around, making it harder to handle the pain.
- You are more likely to need stitches if you have an assisted delivery. The tissues around the birth canal are numb immediately after birth, but if there is any delay in inserting the stitches, ask for a local anaesthetic or gas and air.
- If technology has been used during your labour, the natural mechanism of birth is disrupted. It may be safer to have an injection to make your uterus contract and expel the placenta quickly.

It is policy in some hospitals to speed up labour if you dilate more slowly than would be expected of the 'average' woman (see information on Friedman's curve on page 20). Drips and monitors are waiting in the wings in hospital, so there can be pressure on you to agree to intervention. You might prefer to continue at your own pace, to have nourishing food and some privacy with your partner, or to rest for an hour or two to renew your energy. Ask the midwife if you are not sure whether accelerating your labour is essential or simply an option.

Assisted delivery

Forceps are specially shaped to fit around a baby's head in the birth canal. A ventouse is a small cup that can be fixed with suction.

Normally, the shape of the birth canal, the baby's position and the strength of the contractions ensure that the baby is born in a controlled manner, neither too fast nor too slow. An assisted delivery may help when one or other of these factors is less than ideal.

If your baby's head is tilted, forceps or a ventouse can turn it slightly so that it fits under your pubic arch; if it moves forward and then slides back as each contraction ends, they could hold on, so that your baby makes progress each time you push. They can be used when a baby is premature or in a breech position, to control the speed of the delivery. An epidural may already be in place, or you may have a spinal – a single injection inserted lower down your back.

Caesarean birth

The operation normally takes around an hour to complete and most of the preparations are similar whether you have a local or a general anaesthetic.

Beforehand

Blood samples are taken for cross-matching, and your pubic hair is clipped or shaved. You may have a suppository to empty your bowels, antibiotics to reduce the risk of infection (which can be as high as one in five), and an antacid to neutralise stomach acids. You remove jewellery, contact lenses, make-up and nail polish, so that your colour can be watched during the operation.

A drip to provide fluids or drugs is inserted. Electrodes are taped to your chest to monitor your heart, a blood pressure cuff is put on your arm, and you may be given elastic stockings to help maintain your blood pressure. A diathermy plate, part of the equipment that helps to control bleeding, may be strapped round your leg. Shortly before the operation you may be given extra oxygen to help the baby.

The anaesthetic

Most Caesareans are done under local anaesthetic to avoid the small risks attached to general anaesthesia. Your partner can be present and the excitement of seeing your baby born usually makes up for any nervousness.

An epidural takes thirty to forty minutes to set up, or less if you have one in place that can be deepened. A spinal uses a combination of drugs and is quicker to set up, but it cannot be topped up so an epidural may be set up at the same time in case the operation takes longer than expected and for pain relief afterwards. When the anaesthetic is in place a catheter (a fine tube) is inserted to drain your bladder.

If you prefer not to be awake during an operation, or change your mind at the last minute, you can have a general anaesthetic; lighter gases are used these days so recovery is easier than it used to be.

As you drift off to sleep, a narrow tube is passed into your windpipe and a midwife presses gently on your throat to stop it going down the wrong way. A deeper anaesthetic is given for stitching. Your partner is not usually allowed into theatre during the operation but he can cuddle your baby while you are being stitched.

The operation

An anaesthetist, obstetrician, paediatrician, assistant doctor and two midwives are usually present. If you are awake, your partner sits by your head. A frame with sterile drapes is placed across your chest to block your view.

The incision is usually just below the pubic hair line and is 15–20 cm. long. You may feel as though someone is drawing on your skin with a biro and then rummaging around in a shopping bag. In about ten minutes your baby is lifted above the screen and the placenta is then delivered through the incision.

Tips for Caesarean birth

- Ask if your pubic hair can be clipped instead of being shaved, to avoid the prickly feeling when it grows back.
- If you prefer not to remove your wedding ring it can be covered with tape.
- You could use a personal stereo to mask the normal theatre noises such as taps swishing and instruments clanging, which can sound strange.
- If you feel dizzy or sick you can have extra oxygen or anti-sickness drugs.
- Ask for the screen to be lowered if you want to see your baby being born.
- If you have a general anaesthetic, ask your partner to sit beside you in the recovery room with your baby so that you see them first when you come round.
- Unless there is a crisis, you could ask your midwife to take photos, record your baby's first cries, or help your baby to breastfeed straight after birth.
- You may prefer to wash or shower to reduce the risk of picking up an infection in hospital. Keep your wound dry by patting it gently with paper tissues.
- Take slip-on slippers into hospital, and a wire coat hanger or pair of tongs to retrieve objects that are out of reach.
- Fennel or peppermint tea relieve wind; high-fibre food helps avoid constipation.
- Removing stitches does not usually hurt, but ask for gas and air if it does.
- If you want to go home early, your midwife may be able to remove your stitches or clips; but do make sure that you have plenty of help at home.
- Use a cushion to protect your scar from the seatbelt on the journey home.

Most babies can be cuddled or breastfed during stitching, which takes about forty-five minutes as each layer is repaired separately. The skin is closed with clips or a running stitch with a bead at either end and protected with spray-on film or sticking plaster. A small tube may be left in to drain fluids. Some babies need help to breathe, or special care after a Caesarean birth.

Afterwards

The catheter in your bladder may be removed in theatre or left for several hours. At first you may be given fluids only, then light food such as soup and bread, progressing to a normal diet over a few days. You may have tablets or a heparin injection to reduce the risk of blood clots forming, but will be encouraged to move within twenty-four hours to speed recovery. The scar looks red at first and may weep a little, a natural part of the initial healing process. The usual hospital stay is about five days, or until your stitches or clips are removed.

Pain is generally worst the first day and you may have an epidural top up or an injection, with tablets or suppositories to reduce inflammation. A cocktail of drugs including remedies for wind and heartburn may be offered; or you may have patient controlled analgesia (PCA) where you give yourself pain relief via a machine that prevents overdoses. The drugs are safe for breastfeeding.

Women feel pain differently, but some manage using TENS (with the electrodes placed either side of the scar), the breathing they learned for labour, or homoeopathic remedies such as Raphanus 30 for wind and Arnica 30 for shock to the body. Paracetamol may be sufficient after a few days.

Recovery in hospital

Most women find the first few days after a Caesarean are demanding, but in general, the fitter you are the quicker you are likely to recover.

Moving

To get out of bed, roll on to your side and draw up your knees. Put your top hand on the bed (or against the bedside locker) for leverage and gently swing your body up and your legs down. Ask for a stool if the bed is high.

To stand up, plant your feet apart on the floor. Put both hands on the bed, lean forward and push up. Stand as straight as possible. To walk, slide one foot forward, shift your body until your weight is over it, then slide the other leg forward. Take your time. Use your arms for support when sitting down or getting up. A chair with a high seat and arms may be most comfortable at first.

Breastfeeding

Breastfeeding may take more patience after a Caesarean than after a normal birth. Experiment until you find what is most comfortable – your midwife will help. Lie your baby on a soft pillow over the scar, tuck the baby's legs under your arm in the 'football hold', or lie on your side with her beside you.

Babycare

You will feel wobbly at first and need considerably more help to lift, feed and care for your baby than someone who had a normal birth. Ask whenever you need help. Try to strike a balance between getting mobile gradually, so that you can take on more babycare, and doing so much that you become exhausted.

Choice and control

Where there is trust, there is rarely any conflict, and trust is built rapidly when people are on the same wavelength. If you know the midwife who will help you in labour and have talked about the sort of birth you prefer, she is unlikely to go over your head unless you clearly seem to want this. If she feels something is important she will present the situation in a way that makes it easy for you to make the decision. Most women do not know the staff who care for them, however, and in strong labour women are especially vulnerable; nobody can check out information or argue a point while dealing with powerful contractions.

Choice is important, but too many choices can raise fears and lead to indecision. Sometimes the best choice is to opt out; to do nothing and act on instinct rather than rational decision making. For some women, choosing is fighting. It distracts them from the knowledge that they are perfectly designed to grow babies and give birth to them.

If you want to create a climate where you can remain in charge of your birth, it may help to look at the other side of the coin. Your midwife relies on professional judgement to carry out her job, so while you might worry about having a slow labour speeded up she may feel equally anxious about letting your labour go on for too long without intervening.

You can refuse any treatment, but you cannot force her to treat you in the way you want if it goes against her judgement of the situation. You can decline to have your baby's heartbeat monitored when you first go into hospital, for instance, but you cannot insist on using a birth pool if she refuses because you do not fit the hospital protocol.

People operate best within their individual comfort zones. In practice, you will be able to make any choice you like so long as it falls within the comfort zone of the health professionals caring for you. If not, reasons to deny it will be found: lack of resources, experience or expertise, hospital protocols, research evidence, etc. Your choice will be greatest when your doctor or midwife is sufficiently experienced and confident to have the widest possible comfort zone.

If you have your baby in hospital, you can increase your chances of getting a midwife who is on your wavelength when you phone the hospital before going in. Simply explain the sort of birth you want and ask if you could be assigned someone who would be able to help you to achieve it.

Most health professionals are not out to make you conform to their wishes and neither are you a helpless victim. If a midwife

Dialogue: Discussing treatment

Sarah has had strong contractions for ten hours. She is 4 cm. dilated and she and her midwife feel that everything is fine. The doctor arrives.

Doctor: 'How are you feeling? Your contractions are a bit weak, we could set a drip up to strengthen them.'
Sarah: 'I'm feeling good, thanks. I don't want a drip unless it's essential.'
Dr: 'It's time we got your labour going, this has gone on for long enough. Your baby's fine at the moment but we don't want him to get upset, do we?'
S: 'No, but we're both fine. I'd rather carry on without a drip for now.'
Dr: 'We don't want you to be too tired to push. You're making very slow progress.'
S: 'Are you saying that my labour is abnormal, or that my baby will be in danger unless I have a drip?'
Dr: 'Not exactly, but babies do better if labour doesn't go on too long.'
S: 'I'd like to continue unless it puts my baby at risk. Can we talk about it later?'
Dr: 'OK, another couple of hours, but then we really should make a decision.'
S: 'Thanks, we'll discuss it then.'

Sarah's contractions strengthened naturally after forty minutes and her baby arrived two and a half hours later.

constantly reminds you that all may not go as planned, point out that she is undermining you at a time when you need to be positive and believe in yourself. You know you can change your mind and it will be disappointing, but she must trust you to be flexible. If you find it hard to discuss your treatment or question a procedure, it may help to

---

Dialogue: Challenging intervention

Bryony and Jeff go to hospital to have their third baby. Their other children were born in a midwifery unit, but they have since moved to another town.

Midwife: 'Just hop into bed and we'll hook you up to the monitor for a while.'
Bryony: 'I don't want to be monitored, thank you.'
Mw: 'Everybody has it here. We like to get a base reading of the baby's heartbeat.'
B: 'I didn't have one when my other children were born. It's not essential, is it? Could I have a floor mattress, please, and a birth ball if you have one?'
Mw: 'It's not essential, but we do like to know that your baby is all right at this hospital. It will only be for twenty minutes, then you can do what you like.'
B: 'Thanks, but I don't want it. Just record in my notes that I refused.'
Jeff: 'Could you get a floor mattress? She wants to concentrate on the contractions.'
Mw (providing a small, plastic-covered mattress): 'I have to take your blood pressure and examine you, Bryony. Will you let me do that?'
Jeff (helping Bryony to kneel on the mattress): 'Could you examine her where she is, please? She won't want to lie on the bed.'
Mw: 'I'll do my best – she's in charge, you know!'

---

review some of the sections in Chapter 5 on creating a dialogue.

A doctor or midwife usually appears self-assured when they meet you and you can set the tone for what follows by greeting them equally confidently, head up, hand outstretched, looking directly at them with a smile. You ask questions in order to get the information you need to make a decision, not to cast doubt on their expertise, so assume that they will be happy to answer them.

You do not need to be an expert to ask questions such as:

- Is this procedure (treatment) essential, or is it just an option?
- Will it be safe for my baby if I do (or do not do) this?
- Can you explain the disadvantages as well as the advantages of what you are suggesting?
- Could my partner and I have a few minutes to think about this, please?

Changing your mind

Getting something right is more important than the mild embarrassment of admitting that you were wrong. It can be hard to stay on course and remain positive if the birth cannot be as you wanted, but changing your mind is a privilege to be guarded jealously.

Sticking to a decision has been considered a virtue for generations and it is rarely questioned, but experience can and should shape decisions. Flexibility, adapting to circumstances and trusting your instinct can be positive choices.

Janice: I could have managed to cope with the pain if it hadn't been such a long birth. My labour started one evening and went on all the next day. The second night, I had a sleeping tablet and eventually, almost hysterical with exhaustion, I accepted some pethidine. The next morning, still short of sleep and desperate for help, I had an epidural. I knew I couldn't cope any longer.

With hindsight, I was tense about making the decision and put it off longer than I should have, but once I'd changed my mind it was a relief. Finally, I managed to doze for a few hours, which made all the difference. The birth was fantastic, a really satisfying experience. I was disappointed about having drugs as I'd hoped everything would be normal; but in the long run, it really didn't matter.

Diana: My first labour was induced. The midwives kept giving me a pessary and then apologising a few hours later because they were short of staff and couldn't continue the induction. After two nights without sleep I was distraught. On the third day I had a drip, an epidural and a forceps delivery.

I couldn't face going through it again so I wanted an elective Caesarean this time. My midwife supported me, but when my waters leaked two weeks early she suggested waiting to see what happened. In the middle of the night contractions started and I knew instinctively that I would have a normal birth. I went with my gut feeling, met my midwife at the hospital, and six hours later Rosa was born naturally. I've no idea why I changed my mind, but it felt totally different this time round.

In brief

- The way your labour goes depends on your body type, your emotional state and your baby's position. You can make it easier by staying as relaxed as possible so that your uterus can work with its maximum efficiency.
- If it is your first birth, try not to take labour too seriously too soon. Do whatever takes your mind off your contractions. Sleep if possible – the contractions will wake you when you need to deal with them.
- You do not have to please other people. If you understand the birth process and believe in yourself you will be glad of help when necessary, but not be dependent on doctors or midwives to solve the challenges of a normal life event.
- This is the day of your baby's birth. However it turns out, welcome the experience.

Quick Guide: Is it labour?

A 'yes' to these questions may help you judge if you are in labour:

- Do your contractions keep coming if you change what you are doing – relax in a bath if you were pottering, for example, or walk about if you were resting?
- Are they longer, stronger or more frequent than they were half an hour ago?

If you are still unsure try this test – the closer your score is to '8', the more likely that you are in labour:

- When you change your activity do your contractions:
  Fade away (score 0);
  Stay the same (score 1);
  Get stronger (score 2).
- Your mother or a friend phones to see how you are. Do you:
  Chat away happily (score 0);
  Talk, but break off whenever you have a contraction (score 1);
  Ask your partner to get her to call later as you can't talk (score 2).
- Your partner jokes to keep your spirits up. Do you:
  Appreciate his efforts and laugh (score 0);
  Smile when a contraction finishes (score 1);
  Feel your sense of humour has totally deserted you (score 2).
- Your partner suggests phoning your midwife or the hospital. Is it:
  Too soon, you are perfectly happy (score 0);
  OK, but you are coping well (score 1);
  The right time as you need some support (score 2)?

Quick Guide: Natural birth

	What happens	*How you may feel*	*What to do*
Pre-labour phase	Irregular contractions lasting twenty to thirty seconds and coming five to twenty minutes apart; may disappear when you change your activity.	Excited and bubbly; or sick with stage fright.	Conserve energy: rest or sleep if possible; keep occupied and ignore them.
Early labour	Regular contractions lasting forty-five to fifty seconds; five to ten minutes apart.	Calm and powerful; or edgy and fearful.	Consciously relax and breathe through contractions; pace yourself; try not to take it too seriously too soon.
Strong labour	Frequent contractions, sixty to ninety seconds long, three to five minutes apart.	Deeply calm; or over-whelmed and pushed to your limits.	Breathe slowly; welcome strong contractions (they dilate you faster); look forward to the calm space between them.

	What happens	*How you may feel*	*What to do*
Transition	Irregular contractions, forty to ninety seconds long, two to six minuts apart.	Spaced out or full of energy; or fearful, angry or exhausted.	Take gas and air or kneel with your bottom in the air to help relieve pressure and stop yourself pushing if you are not fully dilated. If you have no contractions or urge to push, stay upright, rest and be grateful; they will start again shortly.
Birth	Contractions last about forty-five seconds and come every few minutes.	Full of energy and confidence; or vulnerable and afraid.	Push towards the burning sensation to numb the tissues as your baby's head crowns.

Quick Guide: Emergency birth

It is unlikely that you will have to deliver your partner's (or your own) baby even if a previous birth was fairly fast but, if it happens, here is how to cope:

- **Don't panic! If your baby is coming quickly, the birth will almost certainly be normal and straightforward.**
- Phone for help if you have time. If not, use common sense: for example, put towels down on a hard or cold floor and get a duvet or blanket for warmth afterwards.
- Stay with your partner and reassure her (and yourself) that all will be well.
- Once the baby's head is born, the body usually tumbles out within minutes. If it does not, feel inside for the cord and gently ease out enough to loop over the baby's head.
- The baby will be wet and slippery. Hold him firmly, angled so that fluids can drain out of his mouth. Wipe away any obvious mucus.
- Leave the cord – it will provide oxygen for several minutes while your baby starts to breathe. The doctor or midwife will see to it when they arrive.
- Cuddling or breastfeeding the baby will help the uterus to contract effectively.
- Keep mother and baby warm by putting the duvet or rug around them both. Some babies are shocked to arrive so fast.
- As soon as your baby is breathing, phone for help if you were unable to do so before the birth.
- A toddler will take everything in his or her stride if you appear calm. Send an older child to phone for help or fetch a neighbour if necessary.

Don't panic! Common sense is more useful.

8

After birth

Good slogans for post-birth recovery are 'look after yourself' and 'give yourself a break'! In the weeks after giving birth, very few women can sustain a high-powered lifestyle without an army of helpers in the background. You may manage to be superwoman on the odd occasion or in short bursts, but the woman who can keep it up day after day usually has plenty of help, an easy-going baby and no other worries. In other words, she is the exception rather than the rule.

It takes nine months to grow a baby, so allow yourself nine months to recover. It may not take that long, depending on your individual make-up, how the birth went and whether you are breastfeeding or not; but it will be several months before all your hormone levels settle down and your body resumes its pre-pregnant state. Meanwhile, you have to adjust to the needs and demands of a small baby. By allowing yourself nine months to get back to normal, you can avoid the stress of chasing an unrealistic goal.

You have gone through the physical and emotional changes of pregnancy, the turmoil of labour or the shock of major surgery, and the exceptionally rapid changes of the first week after birth. With the delivery of the placenta, the factory that produced hormones to maintain your pregnancy shuts down completely. The progesterone

levels in your blood fall and your pituitary gland rel
to tell your body to produce milk. This hormone n
relaxed and switches on maternal behaviour; it also d
sexual arousal and stops ovulation, so indirectly it p
baby by making another pregnancy less likely.

Among all the talk of colic and crying, of pain and problems and sleepless nights, nobody can prepare you for the joy that a baby brings, the bursts of pride you feel as you watch a new life unfold towards you. These feelings are unimaginable and irreplaceable. Relax and enjoy your baby; this special phase lasts for only a few months of your life.

The growth of love

Immediately after a good birth experience you may feel elated, experiencing a rush of emotion higher than any you have ever known. Bathed in birth hormones and the triumph of achievement, blind to puffy eyes, blotchy skin or bruising, captivated by your baby, you are instantly primed for a long-lasting love affair.

Not everyone is so fortunate, however. Even after a straight-forward birth you may be secretly disappointed at the way your baby looks, or proud of yourself, relieved that the birth is over, but rather wary of the baby. If you had a difficult birth, or were distressed by what happened during labour, you may feel detached, desolate or overwhelmed instead of elated. Whatever your experience, you may find it constructive to debrief the birth with the people who helped you.

Great emphasis is placed on bonding, the process of attachment that makes you put someone else's needs before your own; but after either a normal birth or a Caesarean, hormones help you to fall in love with your baby, provided you are given the space and freedom to get to know her in your own way and your own time.

Bonding may take a little longer if the birth was physically diffi-cult or stressful emotionally and you had to suppress your feelings in order to cope; the body and spirit need time to heal. It may also longer if you are separated from your baby through illness, or if you missed out on mothering when you were an infant.

Bonding is not one more thing for mothers to worry about, however; instead, the emphasis placed on it should serve as a reminder to other people not to come between you and your baby unless it is absolutely essential. The quality of the time you spend with your baby can help the process, but it may not happen instantly or even over a few days.

The road to recovery

Within a day or two of giving birth your body may feel as if it has just run a marathon, and you may have a disturbing sense of anti-climax. These feelings often coincide with going home from hospital.

You may be surprised at how bruised, sore and fragile you feel, but your body has gone through quite an upheaval so it is hardly surprising. Common post-natal problems do not always need medical help. Many women use self-help, complementary therapies (see Quick Guide, pages 194–5), or treatments such as Indian head-massage, reflexology or acupuncture to give them a boost post-natally.

Bruising and soreness

Even those who have no stitches usually feel tender or bruised around the vulva for a few days and find walking uncomfortable. Pelvic floor exercises help to disperse swelling, even if you feel very little sensation. For bruising, try homoeopathic Arnica (from pharmacies); or apply Arnica cream if your skin is unbroken. Most women heal quickly after giving birth because the placenta boosts the immune system towards the end of pregnancy.

Lochia

The post-birth discharge lasts for two to six weeks, occasionally longer. It is bright red at first, like a heavy period with small clots, and it is often more profuse during breastfeeding. As it diminishes it turns reddish brown, light brown and finally pinkish. Use sanitary towels rather than tampons to reduce the risk of infection and tell your midwife if it is very profuse or offensive.

It is normal for the lochia to become bright red for a few hours once you are up and about, or whenever you are more active. Each episode usually gets shorter, but the best treatment is to ease up for a while. If you are breastfeeding, your periods may not return until you wean your baby; but if you are bottle-feeding, heavier bleeding four to six weeks after the birth could be a normal period.

Afterpains

These painful cramps, similar to the contractions of early labour, help shrink your uterus to its normal size and expel the lochia. They tend to be worst on the second day. You may barely feel them with a first baby but they get stronger with each subsequent baby. They peak when you breastfeed and diminish as each day passes.

You could take paracetamol or treat them as labour contractions and breathe through them. Homoeopathic Arnica or Mag Phos, or a herbal remedy such as two tablets of cramp-bark three times a day, or tincture of motherwort may help. If they are severe or are still there after a week, tell your midwife so that she can rule out a possible infection.

Sore stitches

A graze or small tear may heal naturally and should feel better in about a week. A larger tear or an episiotomy may take two weeks, and a Caesarean wound will take a little longer to be comfortable. To avoid picking up an infection which could prolong healing for several weeks, pay special attention to hygiene in hospital. Tell your midwife if pain persists or gets worse.

If you had a tear or episiotomy, a bidet or a shower on low power can relieve the stinging from urine; or pour a paper cup of warm water over the area. Ice packs (a bag of frozen peas wrapped in a towel, or a sports-injury gel pack), or bathing the area in hot and cold water alternately, may help with pain. Failing this, ask for treatment from a physiotherapist. Push a rolled-up towel into one leg of a pair of tights and tie it in a ring to relieve the pressure if sitting is uncomfortable. With any scar, if you feel something is not quite right after a few weeks, talk to your doctor.

Sore breasts or nipples

When your milk comes, on about the third or fourth day after the birth, your breasts may become hard, hot and swollen. To relieve this, try bathing them with either hot or cold water; or put dark-green cabbage leaves inside your bra, changing them when they go limp.

Nipple pain caused by 'milk rush' at the start of a feed generally stops after a week or two. If you feel pain throughout the feed, check your baby's position: you should see sucking movement in the jawbone or ear if she is latched on properly. Some babies need patient coaxing to get it right. To ease soreness, smear a paste of slippery elm bark and water on half of a piece of muslin, fold it over and place it inside your bra; or try comfrey root ointment, Calendula cream or Hypercal cream.

Baby blues

This weepy, miserable or fragile feeling is common in the first week after the birth, but it only usually lasts for a few hours or a day or two. You may find yourself becoming over-sensitive or miserable two or three days after the birth, as your milk comes and your body adjusts to different levels of hormones. Typically, women feel tearful or overreact to situations – such as a temporary feeding problem – which they would normally take in their stride. They need support and understanding until they feel stronger (see also Quick Guide: Post-natal illness, page 196).

Post-Caesarean recovery

Going home after a Caesarean can be daunting. You may be distressed at how weak you feel and how much rest you need. Some women cannot even move without help, let alone lift a baby or cuddle a toddler; others appear to recover rapidly only to relapse a few weeks later when lack of sleep kicks in.

At first the scar will look lumpy and red, but over a few weeks it darkens, turns pink and fades to a silvery line covered by your pubic hair. A raised or crooked scar seems to shrink as it heals from the edges. Some women become increasingly upset by the appearance of their scar.

Others lose confidence in their body and feel they cannot take it for granted any more; or they feel fine until a friend has a normal birth several weeks later and it suddenly hits them how disappointed they are to have missed out on the normal birth experience (see Reflecting on the birth, page 186).

It takes some time to get back to normal after any delivery, let alone a birth involving major abdominal surgery. You are more likely to run out of steam rapidly at first, so that having a visitor or going for even a short walk wipes you out for the day. The uterus usually heals completely in about six weeks, but while it does so you will need help with anything that pulls on the wound: lifting, vacuuming and loading the washing machine, for example. Your car insurance may not cover you to drive for six weeks.

How long your recovery takes will depend on how fit you are and whether there were any complications, but as a rough guide:

First week: The wound is painful. You feel weak and need help to lift, breastfeed and care for your baby.
First month: A few women feel physically recovered; most still feel below par. Bending, lifting or lying in certain positions may be uncomfortable, but if the wound hurts a lot or is getting worse, tell your GP.
Three months: Some women have fully recovered, but many still tire easily or lack energy. Pubic hair has grown back to hide the scar.

Six months: Most women have recovered physically. The scar has faded and any twinges or numbness have disappeared.

One year: The majority of women feel fit and well, but a few still feel physically or emotionally unfit; or their scar is still itchy or has numb patches.

Post-Caesarean tips

- Wear loose clothes with pockets to carry things and waist-high pants that do not rub your scar; if the scar itches, keep baby lotion in the fridge to soothe it.

- Duplicate sleeping and nappy-changing arrangements up and downstairs to save energy. Change nappies on a table or chest of drawers to avoid bending.

- Stock up on basics so you do not have to push a supermarket trolley; or order over the phone or on the Internet and pay the small delivery charge.

- To keep up your energy, have a drink and a snack beside you before starting to breastfeed. Leave juice and nourishing snacks in every room so they are instantly to hand; use a thermos flask for hot drinks.

- Delegate as much as possible and accept every offer of help. An extra pair of hands can be well worth the outlay, especially if you have other children.

- If you lose confidence in your body, be honest with your partner. You may need reassurance before you are ready to enjoy sex again.

- List specific jobs for your partner if he is not sure how to help. For example, ask him to load the washing machine before work each day and a neighbour to unload it and hang the washing out.

- Most women find the appearance of their scar improves over time, but if you are unhappy after a few months see your GP.

Caesarean recovery when you have a toddler

- If you are having an elective Caesarean, teach your toddler before the birth that lifting him will hurt your tummy after the baby arrives. Help her to climb into her high chair, fetch a stool to get in the bath and climb in and out of her cot from a chair beside it while you stand nearby. Most toddlers like to be independent.
- Get some new videos to keep her occupied.
- A Caesarean can be an ice-breaker. If your partner drops your child at nursery other mums may offer to bring her home, even if they do not know you well.
- See if your mother or another relative can take some holiday to help out. Make friends with your partner's mother; she may be a gem when you need her.

Relationship strains

The first few weeks after birth can be like the sickness of early pregnancy: stressful at the time, but not without end. You may be caring for a baby who does not know night from day and life may seem to be a series of random collisions – love with fear, pride with self-doubt. Everyone offers advice, but nothing fits together neatly and the learning curve is steep. It can all be rather overpowering.

If you had a difficult birth it is even more important that you and your partner support each other in the days that follow. Give yourselves plenty of time to recover.

Even a normal delivery can be upsetting for a man unless he knows what is happening and feels able to help. Things that are routine for the staff and seem trivial to you at the time can have a major impact on him.

An assisted delivery, or an emergency Caesarean where there is no time to explain what is happening, can be a traumatic experience for everyone, however well prepared. Your partner may try to appear positive and confident while feeling both powerless and terrified for you and the baby. After the birth he is likely to be exhausted, drained of emotion and in need of reassurance.

Some men take on the role of sturdy oak, appearing to be strong when they actually need support themselves. They may worry about the long-term effects of a difficult birth on you and your baby; occasionally they feel so upset that it affects the relationship, perhaps causing conflict over sex or whether to have another baby.

Some people find it hard to talk about a distressing experience while others find talking a relief. It depends on what feels right for the individual. If you want to talk about your experience while your partner does not it is worth bringing this into the open to avoid conflict between you. Many women talk the birth through with their midwife, antenatal teacher or a sympathetic friend.

Most fathers expect, and are expected, to be supportive, but life changes for them as much as for mothers when a baby arrives. They need time to work out their place in the family and sometimes they find the adjustment difficult. If your partner feels he is falling apart he may suffer depression, be irritable, anxious or sleep badly, but he might show it differently, by drinking too much, being aggressive or antisocial, or taking on more work to mask his empty, disconnected feelings.

Exhaustion fuels depression and the body cannot heal itself without rest; it will help your relationship if you make this a priority in the weeks after the birth.

Sleep deprivation

Sleep is associated with health and energy so everyone feels shortchanged when they do not get enough. If your parents made a fuss of you when you were tired as a child, sleep may be a promise of pleasure; if they set great store by it, never allowing you to stay up late for special occasions, missing out may feel threatening.

Sleep disturbance only becomes a problem if it seriously disrupts your life, however, so that you are exhausted every day or so sleepy that it affects your activities. You do not need unbroken nights to get enough sleep because several short bursts can make up for one long session; but you do need extra rest if you are losing sleep regularly. If you wake twice a night to feed your baby and lose an hour's sleep, that is the amount of extra rest to aim for next day.

Your basic sleep rhythm and how much you need for comfort is laid down before birth. Normal sleep blends with the circadian rhythms of your body, which vary over twenty-four hours. They dip between 3 and 4 a.m. (just the time you are woken by a hungry baby) and again at mid-afternoon. If you are already short of sleep, you may hardly be able to keep your eyes open; an early warning that you need more rest.

Research shows that an extra hour's sleep at night eliminates the afternoon dip, but a ten-minute catnap works just as well. Cuddle up with a book on the settee, or use a cot or playpen for your baby if you snooze. Catnaps take practice, but the skill of switching off body and mind is invaluable for catching up after a broken night, or for getting back to sleep at night (see Relaxation, page 129).

Everyone has their own natural energy level and most people sleep badly when overtired. To catch up after one disturbed night, your body needs only a third to half of the sleep missed as it goes straight into deep sleep for a couple of nights, reducing light and dreaming sleep. After two or three broken nights you may not feel on top form; but your long-term health will not suffer. When you are exhausted you will sleep, and after you have caught up you will build reserves to carry you over the next phase of stress or short-term sleep deprivation.

You may want to make as little fuss as possible over night feeds, giving your baby just enough to satisfy her so she does not get used to feeling full in the middle of the night; and not changing her nappy at night unless it is clearly essential! If your baby is fretful, try cutting down on tea and coffee – the stimulants they contain pass into breast milk.

Feeding on demand is easy at first, but it does not have to go on for ever. Within two to three months, many babies can be

A better night's sleep

- Consider replacing an uncomfortable bed – you will spend a lot of time in it.
- Some people find that a twenty-minute walk before going to bed helps them sleep.
- Sleeping well may be better for your relationship than sleeping together. Try alternate nights with your partner, or weekdays apart and weekends together.
- Adjust your bedclothes or open a window to get the temperature right for you and have a bottle of water and some biscuits beside the bed for snacks.
- Unsatisfactory sex can lead to sleeplessness. If you are too tired to enjoy it at the end of the day discuss a better time with your partner.
- Avoid meaningful discussions with your partner before bed-time! Rehearsing scenarios or worrying can stop you sleeping.
- Keep a notebook and pen to jot problems down. Tell yourself, 'I will deal with this at the right time.' It is easier to set time aside for this once you have identified a problem and written it down.
- If you are getting a reasonable night's sleep, check with your GP that you do not have a thyroid problem or anaemia which could be making you tired.

encouraged to space out daytime feeds and drop night feeds. Set yourself flexible targets – distract your baby for half an hour if she wakes early for a feed, and at night, wait for ten to twenty minutes to see if she goes back to sleep, or try to settle her without a feed. A colicky or otherwise high-maintenance baby often becomes more settled at around twelve to sixteen weeks.

You can take a physically demanding job in your stride if you pace yourself, have a break every so often and get just enough sleep to restore your energy. If you ignore your body's signals for too long, however, physical weariness may turn into emotional tiredness.

The answer is to get more rest, but some women find this hard. If your parents were always busy when you were a child, you may feel unproductive and guilty when you are idle. If they valued willingness you may take on extra responsibilities because you feel that 'I'm too tired' is not a good enough excuse for refusing them.

The treadmill becomes an effort, so you do less and feel worse. Your fitness level drops and you become more tired. This sort of exhaustion is a genuine feeling, but it is fuelled by the mind and not relieved by more rest. It makes you feel hopeless and helpless and is often linked with boredom, anxiety or depression.

Black clouds

Admitting to feeling low can be especially hard if you are the sort of person who is generally on top of things, or if your religious or cultural beliefs make you feel that being a 'good enough' mother is never quite good enough. It is easy to accept feelings of stress or depression as your own problem when actually it may be caused by the behaviour of other people: a baby who cries excessively, or getting too little help from your partner, for example.

If unresolved guilt, anger or disappointment linked to your birth experience is preventing you from enjoying life, the sooner it is sorted out the better. Some people discover their own ways to achieve this; others find that professional help given at the right time prevents negative feelings dragging on for months.

While you cannot force yourself to feel differently, you do not want to drift into a cloud so black that you cannot see the way out. Once you know something is not right take your symptoms seriously and seek help without waiting in the hope that it will sort itself out (see Quick Guide: Post-natal illness, page 196).

You are not mad, or a failure, or a bad mother. You are not an inadequate soul who ought to get a grip on herself. You do not deserve to feel the way you do. You just need help. Everyone needs help at times.

Could a professional help?

If you have tried self-help without success, consider seeking professional advice. For each symptom choose the relevant answers and add up your score.

How often is it a problem?
a) Every day, or all the time.
b) Once or twice a week.
c) Once a month, or occasionally.

How much does it affect you?
a) It affects everything I do.
b) It only bothers me at the time.
c) It rarely spoils my enjoyment of life.

How long has it been going on?
a) For several weeks or months.
b) For about two weeks.
c) It has only just started.

Score: a = 5; b = 3; c = 1.
The closer your score is to 15 (the maximum) the more likely you are to benefit from expert advice.

Reflecting on the birth

Taking control can be empowering, but you take control of the whole lot: the pain and the joy, the bad as well as the good. In a strange way it can be as disorientating to achieve the birth you wanted as it is to have your hopes dashed. It takes away the excitement of anticipation: your dream came true, so what next?

When your birth is a disappointment, however, you lose your hopes and expectations and, along with them, confidence and perhaps some self-esteem. Some women are so glad that their baby is healthy that they suppress their anger or disappointment about what happened. Months later, when a friend has a lovely birth or they are pregnant again, they suddenly realise how cheated and upset they feel that they did not have the birth they wanted.

Like any other loss, the pain of disappointment has to be felt and worked through until you can accept the experience and move forward. Nothing can guarantee that a birth will be normal. You can make plans and hold dreams, but your body or your baby may have other ideas.

Some women blame themselves for letting others take decisions for them, but however assertive you are normally, in labour you are vulnerable and the balance of power is weighted in favour of professional opinion. Unless a doctor or midwife includes you it can be hard to challenge their decision. It is unfair to blame yourself for not standing up to them. Give yourself credit for doing your best in the circumstances. Nobody can change the culture of a hospital single-handedly while huffing through contractions in the middle of labour!

Others feel they should have been more flexible, but this is not always as easy as it sounds. Your brain knows that the best-laid plans should change in the light of events, but your heart doggedly struggles on when faced with the situation you wanted to avoid. Dreams are hard to give up.

You may feel upset or angry that the staff did or failed to do something, but people can only make decisions with the information available to them at the time. The best course of action is not always clear except with hindsight. What genuinely seemed best at the time may have turned out to be wrong, but you never know the pitfalls you might have faced if a different decision had been made.

A disappointing experience may have little to do with how you handled labour; it may be nobody's fault and nobody's failure. The answer to the question, 'Why did this happen to me?' may be, 'You drew the short straw, as anyone might have.'

So what happened?

Most women need to understand exactly what took place and why in order to deal with the emotions it produced. Learning from a disappointing experience can turn it into something positive; by understanding exactly what happened you are more likely to be able to file it away and get on with enjoying life. Explanations may lie in the shape of your pelvis, your baby's position, or some well-intentioned intervention that led to an unforeseen problem. Someone may have failed you, the system may have let you down, or you may have unwittingly set yourself up to fail.

If you are not offered a debriefing session before you leave hospital after a complicated or traumatic birth, you could ask for one. Going through what happened so that you understand the reasons for it may set your mind at rest or help you to come to terms with the experience. If you feel upset, angry or let down by someone's attitude, however, even thinking about the birth may be unbearable. You may just want to get on with looking after your baby. It could be several weeks before you feel ready to seek answers or deal with your experience.

It is tempting to keep putting it off and get on with life but, in the long term, knowing what took place and feeling that your distress has been acknowledged can help you to put an experience behind you. As soon as you feel able, ask the hospital for a meeting and for a copy of your notes (see Making a complaint, page 190). These say what happened at the birth, which could help those giving you advice in the future.

You can request a copy of your notes or a meeting to discuss your birth at any time, even many months after the birth. Ask to see a midwife who can explain, or make an appointment with your consultant.

Hearing your side of the story can make a doctor or midwife aware of how devastating an authoritarian attitude or unguarded comment can be, so that they avoid causing distress to other women. Anyone can make a mistake or wish with hindsight that they had bitten their tongue or made a different decision. It takes honesty and acceptance on all sides when there are lessons to be learned, but it means that something valuable can be taken from a negative experience.

Health professionals who face criticism sometimes find it hard to see the issue from anyone else's point of view, however. Confident of their stance or nervous about being sued if they admit to any shortcomings, they are sometimes defensive or they try to soothe you without really listening to what you are saying.

If you worry about being fobbed off with vague reassurance when you want information, take a list of questions: aim to get answers which will help your future decisions. Turn to the section on assertiveness (page 120) before your meeting. Think about your body language: people may misinterpret your feelings if you make self-deprecating statements or have a cheery smile on your face.

If something goes wrong during birth everyone is devastated. Parents feel that the professionals did not take the right action; staff blame themselves for not insisting that their advice was taken. The simple truth is that if there had been a clear indication of what was to come everyone would have acted differently. It is only with hindsight that situations become cut and dried.

Part of getting over a bad experience is accepting that you may never get over it completely; and that while you can move forward, nobody can turn the clock back or wave a magic wand. Ultimately, you have to come to terms with the way the birth was for you.

The learning curve

If your birth was disappointing, your next labour will be a new beginning, a different experience, a chance to learn from the past without allowing it to dictate the future. You have to find your own answers, but you could start by looking at anything you feel was a mistake in your last birth. See it as a learning opportunity so that it does not happen again.

Ask a close friend who has children to explain what she would do differently another time, or what she felt helped her. She may claim she was lucky if her birth was good, or praise someone else if it was difficult; but probe deeper: how did she create her luck, choose her midwife or birth partner, manage her fears?

If you had a difficult or disappointing experience, you may need extra support when you have another baby, but a subsequent birth which goes well can be the best healer of all. In dealing with your previous experience you have become a stronger person and gained self-knowlege. Use this awareness.

You may know more about your partner, the services available and how to steer your way through them. You may have learned not to leave things to chance, to value your instinct or to ask more questions. You may be able to define your goal more realistically, taking account of what is best for you and your baby instead of clinging to a dream.

Sometimes, it takes more than one birth to achieve what you want because you simply do not have the knowledge you need; or the child in you is fearful and needs to summon up the courage to take necessary action. Once you are ready to let go, a barrier often disappears; and with the resolve not to leave it all to chance you are in a better position to achieve the birth you want next time round.

Handling disappointment

- You are not wrong to feel upset or disappointed: feelings are not right or wrong, they simply express an emotion that exists.
- Find someone who will listen and accept how you feel, not brush aside what you say. It can take time and several attempts before you find the words you need to express your experience and how you feel about it. Keep trying.
- Try not to blame yourself for being unrealistic about labour – everyone learns some things the hard way. Self-criticism only makes it harder to let go of fear.
- Find a good midwife or antenatal teacher to help and support you if you have another baby. You have the right to hold a dream and to rebuild it if you wish.

Making a complaint

Many women do not want to make a formal complaint about their treatment. They simply want to understand what took place. If something distressed them and it could have been avoided, they want this to be taken on board so that it does not happen again.

They want to be treated with respect, given explanations and their feelings to be acknowledged. Sadly, this does not always happen.

Litigation is stressful for all concerned and in nobody's interests if a conflict can be resolved in any other way. If you feel you are getting nowhere, however, or you want to avoid other women having to go through a similar experience, you may consider making a formal complaint. It can be a wearisome job, but it is sometimes the only way to change outdated attitudes and practices, or to right a wrong. Changing what happens in the future can provide some comfort.

Immediately after a disappointing birth many women feel vulnerable and want to put the whole episode behind them. They want to get on with recovering their health and looking after their baby; but if you or your partner feel you might wish to complain at a later date, take action as soon as possible. It does not oblige you to proceed, but it is easier to withdraw a complaint than to initiate one at a later date, when staff may have moved on or deadlines may be close to expiry.

The Health Information Service can advise you further about the procedure; if you need information or support, contact Aims. These are the main steps to take:

- Jot down or tape record every memory of the incident. This is easier soon after the birth than a few weeks down the line.
- Request copies of all your case notes, including those held by your GP and any computerised hospital records for you and your baby.
- Send a preliminary letter saying that you wish to put it on record that you intend to complain about your care and you will detail your complaint in due course.

Your memories

Record as soon and as accurately as possible everything you recall: dates, times, who was there, who said what, how you felt and so on. Ask your birth partner or anyone else who was there to do the same.

Check this against your case notes – the staff concerned may recall events differently.

Case notes

Get your notes before any mention of a complaint comes up. You do not have to say why you want them; occasionally they go mysteriously missing or entries are altered once it is known that a complaint may be made. If you request your notes during pregnancy or within forty days of the last entry in them you only pay for photocopying and postage. After this there may be an administration fee.

Preliminary letter

If you might want to make a complaint at a later date this sets the procedure in motion. You may not feel up to taking it any further until you have had a chance to fully recover after the birth, or to surface from the first few months of looking after your baby, so this preliminary letter is important to avoid the complaint being ruled out of time. Keep copies of all correspondence.

Getting back to normal

Motherhood is rewarding, but the first few months can be challenging so think about your own welfare as much as your baby's. Junk food and exhaustion fuel depression and your body cannot heal itself without sleep. Make resting to catch up on lost sleep a priority. A healthy lifestyle helps you to get back to normal.

- Tea and coffee can limit the absorption of iron, leaving you anaemic. Drink water, fruit juice or herbal teas sometimes. Two cups a day of peppermint tea with a half-inch chunk of fresh ginger root grated into it can be revitalising.
- For a quick pick-me-up, blend a glass of milk with two table-

spoons of natural yogurt and a banana; or a glass of orange juice with six dried apricots (buy them pre-soaked) and a teaspoonful of honey. A teaspoon of brewer's yeast added to each gives extra vitamin B.

- If your diet includes plenty of fruit, vegetables and whole grains such as brown rice and wholemeal bread, you will automatically get nutrients such as vitamins B1 and C, which help combat tiredness.
- Take a brisk walk in the fresh air every day with your baby in a buggy or sling. This can help you to sleep better and it releases hormones that 'lift' your mood.
- Join a group, or keep up with friends by phone, letter or E-mail. Making an effort to find new friends and interests may also help (see Directory, page 215).
- Pace yourself: space out commitments such as lunch with a friend by automatically fixing a date two to three weeks ahead, even if your diary is not full.
- Enjoy your baby, look after yourself and your partner; and give yourself a break.

In brief

- Post-natal aches and pains do not always need medical help; you may want to try self-help or complementary therapies.
- If you think professional advice would help, seek it straight away rather than hoping the problem will go away by itself.
- If your birth experience was disappointing, talk to the staff who cared for you to try to understand the reason for the problem.
- Whatever sort of birth you want you can help yourself and there are people who will help you. If you look back on your birth experience with satisfaction, talk to other women about it. Hearing your story will empower them.

Quick Guide: Complementary therapies

Aromatherapy oils, herbal preparations and homoeopathic remedies are widely available from pharmacies. They can have side effects, so use the smallest recommended dose to see how it affects you and increase it if necessary. If you have any doubts or you are breastfeeding, consult the pharmacist or a qualified therapist. Some remedies are best prescribed individually.

- **Sore stitches**
  Aromatherapy: bathe the area with three drops patchouli or tea tree oil in a bowl of warm water, or add three drops each of lavender and cypress oils to a shallow bath.
  Herbalism: apply Calendula or Hypercal cream directly to the wound; to prevent infection, pour four pints of boiling water on to 4 oz. of dried yarrow, rosemary or witch hazel; leave for eight hours; strain into a shallow bowl and sit in it for fifteen minutes daily.
  Homoeopathy: try Arnica followed by Calendula for five days or alternate doses of Ars Alb and Hepar Sulph. For burning pain, try Causticum 30 twice daily for four days.

- **Depression**
  Aromatherapy: clary sage and bergamot help depression; geranium, grapefruit, mandarin, neroli and rose oils give a mental lift. Use two to three drops (individually or combined) in a burner, four to six drops in your bath, or up to five drops per teaspoonful of vegetable oil for massage.
  Herbalism: drink a cup or two of lemon balm tea with milk and honey every day for two weeks. Blessed Thistle (up to twenty drops of tincture, two to four times a day) may help, or try St John's wort.
  Homoeopathy: try Lycopodium, Calc Carb, Sepia, Kali Phos or Nat Mur.

- **Headaches**

  Aromatherapy: mix one drop peppermint oil, three drops lavender and a drop of any vegetable oil and massage into your temples or the base of your skull; add six drops of each oil to half a pint of water and soak a compress for your forehead.

  Herbalism: make an infusion of equal quantities of lemon balm, lavender and meadowsweet, or drop two cloves into a cup of tea.

  Homoeopathy: remedies for different types of headache include Hypericum, Nat Mur and Kali Bich.

- **Insomnia**

  Aromatherapy: try a drop of lavender, neroli or clary sage on your pillow, or two drops each of chamomile and lavender in a room burner.

  Herbalism: infuse a handful of Californian poppy or elderflower in a pint of boiling water and strain it into a hot bath after thirty minutes; or try a small cup of chamomile tea with milk and honey before bed.

  Homoeopathy: for nervous exhaustion improved by sleep, Kali Phos; or Nelson's Noctura tablets (from pharmacies).

Quick Guide: Post-natal illness

- **Post-natal depression** affects about 10 per cent of women, shortly after the birth, or several weeks or even months later. It is a feeling of being cut off from everyone and unable to help yourself: you may be irritable, cry easily or smile too brightly; be unable to sleep even when your baby sleeps, or be afraid to accept invitations and hide if anyone calls. You may lose interest in life, feel overwhelmed by everyday tasks, or stick to a rigid routine as though it were a security blanket. Talk to your GP if symptoms last for more than two weeks.

- **Anxiety conditions** include panic attacks (your baby's crying terrifies you, for example), compulsive thoughts or actions (cleaning relentlessly for fear of germs), or constant mild anxiety (like butterflies in your tummy) when facing more pressure than you feel able to handle. They can be masked by depression, as emotional distress makes you feel low. If extra support does not relieve the symptoms, ask your GP to refer you to a clinical psychologist for cognitive behavioural therapy.

- **Post-traumatic stress disorder** (PTSD) is linked to suffering excessive pain or to feeling completely powerless, ignored or denied information. Up to 2 per cent of women suffer nightmares, sleep disturbance or flashbacks of birth events. Some women handle it best alone, but if the symptoms last longer than a month, or if it begins to haunt you again when you thought you had got over it, talk to your GP.

- **Puerperal psychosis** is rare, affecting about one woman per thousand. It occurs within days of birth, so hormones may play a part. Typical sufferers are hyperactive or have extreme mood swings, delusions or hallucinations. Your GP will arrange treatment, which may involve a stay in hospital. Most women recover well.

9

Women talking

The women who share their birth stories in this chapter would not describe themselves as outstanding in any way. They have had varying experiences, from the deeply satisfying to the unexpectedly traumatic, but they have in common an inner strength brought out by the birth of their children. Where they could, they took control of their experience; where they could not, they learned from it.

The courage that women bring to the birthing experience never fails to amaze me. They emerge as different people, stronger and more resilient, able to take on the responsibility of nurturing a child. One woman said to me: 'It was a tremendously empowering experience that has helped me to be my son's advocate.' These are their stories:

Letting go

Angela Hopper (33) is a reflexologist and mother of Elsa (2½) and Rosie (3 weeks). During her travels she lived with indigenous people and attended ceremonies celebrating the birth of babies only an hour old. This background helped to form her perception of birth.

'I wanted Elsa's birth to be my own experience, so I relaxed, meditated and read about active birth and water birth. I wasn't frightened; I simply trusted that everything would be all right. The birth process is completely natural and at home it unfolds as it should.

'My partner Gareth was always supportive because he knew I was well-prepared and trusted myself. It wasn't a whim. My GP told me I was mad to want a home birth: if she lived in the country she would move into a hotel near the maternity hospital for two weeks before her due date! I thought that was ridiculous and was determined not to take on board anyone else's fears.

'Most of the midwives seemed to think that I had an over-romantic view of birth and said I should go into hospital to have my first baby, but nobody could give a medical reason for this. Eventually, they respected my choice and supported me.

'The birth was a wonderful experience because I felt in control the whole time. I spent about four hours in the water pool and gave birth to Elsa standing up, holding on to the edge and laughing. It was just how I imagined it and I felt proud that I had trusted myself and not been influenced by anybody. There was ecstasy, utter joy and wonderment because we had done it all ourselves. That feeling lasted for about a year.

'I adored Elsa because she had helped me, worked with me. After everyone had left she started coughing and spluttering and some instinct told me to call an ambulance. As it turned out she was fine; the person who needed emergency treatment was me. I had a blood transfusion and was told that I was very lucky – had I gone to sleep I might have lost consciousness. I felt that Elsa saved my life.

'Rosie's birth was totally different. I came up against more opposition because of the bleeding and a strep B infection. The consultant said I would need intravenous antibiotics during labour and they could not be given at home. I thought, "Here we go again, let's do the research."

'The strep B helpline confirmed that I could have IV antibiotics at home. Then I met a woman who had a home birth with oral antibiotics for strep B and she put me in touch with her consultant who was researching it and felt that oral antibiotics were effective.

My midwife said that this was not the policy at the local hospital and they could not follow his regime without evaluating the research; but eventually they decided the best oral dose for me.

'I seemed to be bombarded by one problem after another. A midwife would be worried about the bleeding I'd had when Elsa was born. The next would say that was no problem, but she was concerned that the baby was big and I might not be able to have a normal birth. It was as though they were conspiring against me.

'I started to get paranoid because everyone except Gareth undermined me. I lost confidence in my body, not because of the bleeding, but because I took other people's anxieties on board. So much was happening that I had no time to relax and get all the niggly worries in perspective. Gareth was caught up with work and neither of us was really able to focus on the birth.

'Elsa had arrived on time. Rosie was a week overdue, then two weeks. The birth pool was sat in the corner of the bedroom, waiting to be filled. Perhaps I was not ready to give birth because of the build-up of stress; or perhaps my instinct was in charge and I was meant to have Rosie in hospital. I had no flicker of doubt about a home birth last time, but this time I felt myself wavering. I couldn't step back and convince myself that everything would be fine, nor imagine having her at home.

'Three weeks after my due date, my waters were broken in hospital. Less than an hour before Rosie was born in the water pool, I was sitting in the hospital garden enjoying the sunshine. She arrived so fast that I felt frozen, frightened and out of control. There was no problem with bleeding afterwards and I recovered very quickly. I just couldn't quite believe that Rosie had arrived.

'The way a birth goes depends partly on how you are in yourself. It's about feeling all right about the whole thing, so that you are able to let go.'

Handling the past

Cindy Herraman-Stowers (35) is a PR executive. She had to overcome traumatic medical experiences in her past in order to have her daughter, Isabella.

'Getting pregnant was a major decision for me and I knew that I would need to avoid too much emotional distress, so it was vital to be well-organised right from the beginning. Before I decided to go ahead, I made an appointment with my doctor in Australia and took along about forty questions about different kinds of birth. I wanted to have a good idea of what each entailed.

'We talked about natural birth, epidurals and Caesarean section. I knew that I couldn't cope with an epidural – when I was fifteen I had a lumbar puncture that was a horrendous experience. If I went for a natural birth I would have worried for nine months that I might end up with an epidural.

'By this time I was pregnant and desperately needed some control over what is basically an uncontrollable situation. I made an appointment to see a doctor who knew me well because she had looked after me for a gynaecological problem. We discussed what my body would be capable of and my feelings about the birth. She recommended an elective Caesarean section under general anaesthetic.

'At this point, my husband Mark and I found we were about to move from Australia to the United Kingdom. I had no idea what would happen there, but my obstetrician knew a GP who lived not far from where we were going. That lucky break saved me having to hunt around for the right contacts once I reached the UK.

'The GP referred me privately to a female obstetrician at the local hospital and I prepared for our first meeting by writing all my questions down, knowing that when I saw her I would be nervous and forget things. My case might have been strong enough to have what I wanted on the NHS, but I was privileged to be able to go private and it probably helped me to have an easier time.

'Once I had decided that having a Caesarean under general anaesthetic was not negotiable, I put across my position and stated my reasons and everyone accepted that I knew what I wanted. The obstetrician agreed to share my care with a local, privately run maternity centre. If she had not been prepared to take me on I would have gone elsewhere, or flown back to Australia to have the baby.

'At a difficult or anxious time, people need privacy and dignity and I wanted Mark to stay with me and build the family unit, so I asked how I should go about getting a private room. Basically, I said this is what I'm looking for and these are my reasons for wanting it; how do I go about getting it? I backed up my decisions with reasons and was never made to feel that I was being silly.

'Everybody was supportive and nobody tried to push me down a road I didn't want to go, so from the outset I had peace of mind. I built a relationship with the obstetrician and the midwives and trusted them to be honest with me but to understand how I felt.

'For the first few months of pregnancy, I still cried at night, thinking about the operation, but I knew what would happen and talked at length about the bits that frightened me. That helped me feel a bit more in control.

'The birth went better than I'd expected and some of the things that I had thought would be distressing from my previous experience, were fine. Isabella was born at 9 a.m. By 6 p.m., they offered to remove my catheter and drip if I really couldn't face them any longer, but I kept them until the following morning, a major achievement for me.

'I stayed one night in hospital and then went to the maternity centre for a few days. There the reaction kicked in and I cried when Isabella was not asleep and then cried with relief when she was!

'Having a baby is a huge achievement for every woman and doing it my way gave us peace of mind. It cost what Mark and I might have paid for a special holiday and it was worth every penny. I coped with my past experience and feel really proud of myself. We laid good foundations for our family to build upon.'

Changing plans

Jane Lamer (29) is a training and development advisor. She was determined not to be sidetracked by anyone, but to give birth the way she wanted.

'During my pregnancy I read widely, visited all the websites, talked to anyone who had had a natural birth and could give me tips and went to antenatal classes. I "interviewed" my midwife with a list of questions. We formed a good relationship, but if she had not been supportive I would have tried to find someone else. Ultimately, I wanted to give birth my way.

'My hind waters broke before Aidan's head was engaged and I was told to go straight to the consultant unit of the local hospital, threatening my plans for a water birth in the midwifery unit. I felt emotional when I arrived and launched with all guns blazing into what I would and would not do! The midwife said gently that she could not force me to do anything against my will and she would not try, so I relaxed and agreed to be monitored for twenty minutes, with my eye on the clock.

'As I was five centimetres dilated and all was well, I asked to transfer to the midwifery unit as planned and she agreed, but after fourteen hours in and out of the water pool, Aidan's head was still high and my cervix was not dilating. I was very upset, but I understood why I needed to return to the main unit.

'I wanted a natural birth and the midwives helped me to try everything possible. They have to follow protocols, so they told me what they wanted to do and I told them whether they could do it or not. I was well able to discuss the options and they were fine about it.

'I did not get everything I'd hoped for, but there were always good reasons and we had a dialogue between equals. I didn't assume they always knew best, but took their advice when it was right for me and for Aidan. They respected my wishes and did it my way as far as possible, because they could see that I had thought about the birth and wasn't being stubborn or unrealistic.

'The doctor who broke my waters expected me to stay on the bed and be continuously monitored. I asked why and he had no answer, so I said, "Can I walk around and can you fetch a birth ball from the midwifery unit for me to use?" He seemed surprised but agreed readily.

'I decided to have an epidural, but even with this and a drip Aidan's head did not engage, so I had a Caesarean. It may not have been what I planned but it was what I wanted in the circumstances and in my heart I knew I needed it. There is no point in fighting against something when the circumstances change.

'For a short while afterwards I mourned not having the natural birth I thought I should have been able to achieve because other, less determined women do; but we did everything possible. At no point in my labour did anything happen that I did not understand. I always felt in control, so it was a genuinely positive experience.

'The key is to be informed and not intimidated by medical staff. It may seem as though you are expected to do as you are told, but when you query things they are fine about it. I did not ask questions to be clever, but because I needed to know.

'I felt the staff respected me because I wanted to know what was going on and that made me feel more comfortable. Even a long labour is not too bad when you are involved in the process and things are not being done *to* you but *with* you.'

Moving forwards

Nicola Comben (26) is an accountant. Her birth was especially traumatic, but she has faced her memories with courage and moved on to enjoy life with her daughter, Emily.

'My family had natural births and I never imagined that mine would be different. Millions of women have babies and I felt in my heart that I could do it. I wanted a natural birth for the baby's sake, but also to share the early memories with my husband Craig and with our parents.

'Craig and I went to antenatal classes, where I focused on preparing for what I wanted, a natural birth. When Caesareans were mentioned the shutters went up. I could not bear to think of missing the early weeks with my baby.

'My contractions started on Tuesday evening. On Thursday morning, I went into the midwifery unit, five centimetres dilated and feeling in control, carried along by excitement. Emily had her back to mine and I progressed one centimetre in four hours so when the midwife suggested breaking my waters I hoped it would get the labour going. Sure enough the contractions came thick and fast.

'All day I focused on getting through each one, unaware of how long it was taking; but the moment the midwife suggested an epidural I wanted one. All my fears about injections in my spine went. When she mentioned the possibility of a Caesarean section, panic rose, but I was willing to do anything to get this baby out vaginally. At last I was fully dilated and I pushed and pushed until Craig could see Emily's head. The registrar then decided to try a ventouse delivery, but it failed and Emily became severely distressed.

'During the emergency Caesarean I felt agonising pain but was too tired and confused to speak properly. I could not even protest. The operation ended a hair's breadth away from a hysterectomy. Afterwards, I thought that I had imagined it and for the first week I kept crying tears of frustration, unable to put my experience into words. Everything felt so unfair.

'My surgeon said he could refer me for counselling, although he did not agree with it. His comment was off-putting, but I felt it was something for me and my family so I swallowed my pride and went. I got a depth of understanding that proved to be a lifeline in the days that followed.

'Counselling helped me to accept that mine was not a normal Caesarean delivery and that I really was very ill after it. From the moment I had the epidural I was thinking only of myself, so I felt guilty about causing Emily the distress of the ventouse delivery. I had to come to terms with this and with my disappointment that the experience did not measure up to my dream of a natural birth.

'I realised that, like many women, I wasn't really open-minded. I had constructed an ideal birth in my mind and that is what I lost.

'My counsellor also helped me to accept that I was angry, and that it was reasonable to feel like that. I would have done anything to have a natural birth, but at the same time the staff let me go on for too long and the anaesthetist did not make sure I felt no pain during the operation. I understand the pressure she was under, but she was responsible for my nightmare.

'I'm still coming to terms with losing the time immediately after the birth. Craig and I wanted a daughter so much and it should have been so perfect, but I was too ill to enjoy it. I see him coming towards me with a dark-haired baby, but I don't even remember how I found out that she was a little girl. I feel cheated that we could not share those precious early memories of our firstborn. We'll never get the start of our family life back again.

'For the first few months, I coped on autopilot. My friends from antenatal classes had good births, maybe not easy but more or less what they wanted. I was devastated, unable even to breastfeed because I was so tired. I missed out on Emily's early development; nine months is a long time in a baby's life.

'My family just kept loving me, letting me express my feelings and accepting them as valid without suggesting that I should just "get over it". I knew my parents would always be there for me; but my soul would have died if it hadn't been for Craig's love.

'Very few women have complications after an emergency Caesarean and some people's attitude is: "You had a Caesarean? You have a healthy baby, get on with your life!" I'm grateful for my lovely daughter, but I could never have been prepared for what happened. I have worked hard to be able to acknowledge the experience and file it away. People say, "You'll be fine, you'll have another baby", but it isn't that easy. I'm getting my life back to normal at present and I need all my energy to get over the experience. I cannot forget and inevitably there are times when I feel sad.

'I don't regret the labour or the birth, even the pain in theatre although I would rather it hadn't happened. With the help of my counselling I can say, "It was hell, but I got through it." I've always wanted a second baby and feel I need to give birth again to get it "right", but there isn't a right way. However hard you try you cannot always have the birth of your dreams; but you can move forward and come through it a stronger person.'

Lessons to learn

Gill Mundham (36), a health visitor for eleven years, was looking forward to having her first baby in the peace and privacy of her own home.

'There was no seed of doubt in my mind about wanting to have my baby at home. When I was a midwife I delivered babies in hospital and at home and you just can't compare them. At home, women are more relaxed, it's like a party with everyone laughing and joking. As a health visitor I spoke to lots of women and nobody had a bad home birth.

'I never worried about how long my labour would last because I'd seen some women deliver in four hours while others took days. They all had healthy babies in the end and at home there is no pressure, so it hardly matters. I was prepared to go into hospital if necessary, but the statistics show that home birth is safe and my midwife was enthusiastic. I felt supported and confident.

'Of course, I did have fears. I worried about handling pain and about the baby lying back-to-back because this was linked in my mind with forceps and Caesarean section. In the end, despite doing all the right things to get Katherine into a good position, she was lying back-to-back. My challenge was to find out if I could actually cope with labour and I proved to myself that I could.

'My waters broke early and the pain was continuous and everywhere, but relaxing in my birth pool at home I imagined myself elsewhere until I was fully dilated. Then my contractions stopped. Katherine's heartbeat was fine and I could even feel her head, but there were no contractions. I tried rest, nourishing food and homoeopathic remedies, but there was no power to help me push.

'My husband Richard drove me into hospital, with one midwife ahead and another behind in case the baby arrived in the car. I was happy to transfer because we'd tried everything and I was so tired that if the contractions came back I wouldn't have had any energy. To be honest, I wanted it over.

'I worried that the staff would criticise my choice of a home birth because a few years ago I might have made such a comment myself; but everyone seemed genuinely sorry that it hadn't worked out for me and that meant a lot to me.

'A drip was set up, but Katherine became distressed. The registrar tried to deliver her by ventouse, then performed an emergency Caesarean section. I was utterly shocked.

'I don't feel that I failed, but I do think that I had lessons to learn. I anticipated not being able to cope with the pain, or going to hospital for an epidural and possibly ending up with an assisted delivery. I never dreamed that I might need a Caesarean. That was for "them", those other women who were too posh to push or whatever. With all my knowledge I still judged people and secretly thought that women who had a Caesarean were taking the easy way out.

'I came home the day after my operation – early by anyone's standards, but the sympathetic registrar made it easy by signing my discharge papers. She wouldn't normally have agreed, but if I'd discharged myself I might have been reluctant to go back had anything happened.

'You learn most from the things that you get wrong; those you get right you take for granted. Had my experience been straight-forward I might have been arrogant about birth. It was horrible at the time, but I moved light years ahead. I wasn't nearly as flexible as I thought; I had to be made to listen and perhaps there was no other way. Now I empathise with women who have a difficult labour and for that alone it was a positive experience.

'I felt empowered throughout my birth, and with hindsight I'm not convinced that Katherine was distressed. Given a bit more time, if I had not been so tired, if there had been someone else there as well as Richard, could I have stuck it out and still have had a normal delivery? If I have another baby I'll need to bury my ghosts, but I will try for a home birth again.'

Finding the right people

Liv Simonsen (31) is an operating department practitioner, trained to assist with operations. She had a breech birth at home, attended by an independent midwife.

'Hospital does not seem to me to be a good place to have a baby. The nurse-patient relationship is never equal; everyone slips into their roles and patients are treated in a way that undermines their ability to speak up for themselves.

'I had no experience of normal birth, having only seen Caesareans, but I chose a home birth because I wanted it to be intervention-free. I thought I would be less likely to get this in hospital because of the culture. Women are vulnerable in labour. They can't argue with anyone about anything and I didn't want to rely on my partner Steve to fight for me. Men are empowered by normal labour and by being a parent, but with the first baby they don't have that experience.

'Very early in pregnancy, before I even saw my GP, I wrote to the supervisor of midwives at my local hospital requesting a midwife for a home birth. I expected opposition as it was my first baby, but there was none. My midwife was not enthusiastic, but although I would have liked someone who was excited about a home birth she was basically there to do a job for me.

'When I was thirty-seven weeks pregnant we discovered that Zachary was breech and, despite all my acrobatics, he looked like staying that way. The midwife said the birth would have to be in hospital.

'Our antenatal teacher gave us a leaflet which said that, except for certain circumstances, the risks of a breech birth are not that high, so I thought about a vaginal birth in hospital. The consultant I was referred to favoured Caesarean section for breech delivery, so I asked around and wrote requesting to see one who sounded more open-minded.

'At my appointment, I was told that home birth was dangerous because midwives do not carry any oxygen or resuscitation equipment! That was incorrect and I said so. I knew from my job that there is no magical equipment for saving babies in hospital. There is nothing that we could not have at home. People can be swayed by inaccurate information.

'The consultant said that I could either have a Caesarean or a vaginal breech delivery with forceps and an epidural. I thought my pelvis would not perform well if I lay flat on my back with an epidural and forceps sounded horrible. I thought that a Caesarean would be less traumatic for me and Zak.

'Then I had a stroke of luck. A friend mentioned an independent midwife who lives nearby and delivers breech babies. It sounded wonderful . . . but we had no money to pay for private care. Nevertheless, we arranged to meet Mary and it was like sinking into a huge, soft armchair. She was so confident. She didn't think having a breech vaginal birth was a problem, or that it was dangerous. She felt I was totally entitled to it, and she said that she would rather deliver a baby for nothing than see someone have an unnecessary Caesarean section.

'The relief was so immense that I still get tearful when I think of it. We could only offer to do things in her garden in return, although later I asked my parents to help and we were able to pay her. Before we met Mary, we were always pushing at the barriers – a midwife who wasn't keen, a consultant dictating how I had to have the baby in hospital. Afterwards, all our concerns drained away. I was enormously pregnant and needed someone to say, "Look, it can be done."

'My waters broke at about 11 a.m., two weeks early. Half an hour later, I was in strong labour. It was not at all what I'd expected and nothing was ready – I thought we'd have plenty of time to go for a walk and cook a nice meal. It was incredibly painful but I wasn't worried at any time. Mary brought some Entonox, but had I been in hospital I'd have asked them to give me everything and missed out on a totally amazing experience.

'I'm proud that I had a breech home birth and so grateful to the midwife who made it possible. There are different theories on every subject and you don't have to accept the first thing you hear. Despite what everyone who supposedly knew better was telling me, I got the birth I wanted by finding the right people to help me. It was a tremendously empowering experience.'

Taking control

Vicky McFarlane (31) is a teacher. Her triumphant first birth helped her to deal with a less positive experience the second time around.

'Before Alistair was born all I knew about birth was what I'd seen on TV: drama where it was horrendously painful, or comedy where it was funny as well as painful, the extremes of the experience.

'When I read about water birth it sounded calm. My aunt is an antenatal teacher and she lent me a video. My husband Ross and I saw this woman doing a couple of huffs and puffs and then giving birth. We looked at each other and said, "It can't be that easy!"

'We had to find out about water birth for ourselves. The midwife said it was not something that she could promote, but she would support whatever we wanted. Once we had decided, she turned out to be very positive about it.

'My birth plan said I didn't want pain-relieving drugs. The first midwife I met when I was in labour read it, huffed and said, "You can always change your mind", which was scary. I thought she must know better than me! But I got into the pool and it was blissful. The birth was just like the video: natural and lovely. I was exhilarated, not exhausted, and the staff made me feel special.

'When I was expecting Abigail, my scan at eighteen weeks showed a low-lying placenta. Nobody seemed to think it would be a problem or stop me from having another water birth. I was told that they'd scan me again later on.

'Then we moved to another area because of Ross's job. The contrast was striking. I was pressured to move from midwife-led to consultant-led care and when the midwife read my notes she said there was no chance of a water birth, I would probably need a Caesarean section because my placenta was low. "Your baby could die and so could you," she said. I was terrified.

'During our hospital tour, another midwife made a throwaway comment which rang alarm bells. She said Caesareans were quite common at that hospital. In a panic I phoned my aunt, who told me how to get the statistics for the hospital. It had one of the highest Caesarean section rates in the UK.

'The placenta was still rather low at my second scan, so I asked friends with a medical background to look things up for me, so that I would be able to discuss it sensibly with my doctor. My aunt put me in touch with an experienced independent midwife who could discuss the need for a Caesarean. She said that if my placenta was closer to my cervix than a certain measurement an operation would be safest, but if not I should be all right. The uterus would draw the placenta further away as it expanded. She suggested asking the radiographer to tell me the measurement.

'After my third scan, I was able to say to the doctor, "My placenta is so many centimetres away from the cervix so that's fine, isn't it? I don't need a Caesarean after all!" Even so, four days before my due date, I was told to think about having the baby induced.

'Finding things out for myself gave me the confidence to resist pressure to have a managed birth. My GP treated me as an equal throughout, but the midwives behaved as though they knew what to do and expected me to conform. Had I not had such a different experience with my first baby, I might have felt that was how it had to be done and who was I to question anything?

'When I went into hospital in labour, people kept popping their head round the door, asking things like, "Do you need any more rubbish bags?" A private experience was turned into a public spectacle.

'The midwives kept making excuses as to why I couldn't have a water birth, each giving a different reason: the birth pool was free but they were too busy at the moment; it hadn't been cleaned, but they would sort it out; someone was still using it; and so on. I knew I was being fobbed off, but I didn't have the energy to argue. I feel angry with myself, but Ross and I were freaked out by the "problem" of my placenta. Neither of us felt in a strong position.

'Abigail's birth wasn't awful but, mentally, it wasn't as rewarding as Alistair's. The staff did it their way rather than mine and that took something away from me. When Alistair was born I lifted him out of the water. I was the first to see him and to know that he was a boy. It was a brilliant experience. I was glad the midwives were standing by, but I didn't need them. They empowered me to deliver him myself.'

A personal journey

Clare Burt (27) had an emergency Caesarean with Emma (6) and an elective Caesarean with Lucy (4). Jack (6 months) was born naturally at home.

'When Emma was born after a difficult labour, I felt my body had let me down. I was just twenty-one and it was all good fun, a bit of a laugh, until the birth started to go wrong. Then it was a roller-coaster and Jason and I didn't know how to cope.

'Jason works in the family business and his parents had booked a special holiday not knowing that it would coincide with Emma's birth. He was left in charge. With hindsight, he could have shut the business down for a week, but he felt he had to battle on. I've always needed a bit of a cheering squad and I didn't get that support when I was in labour with Emma.

'I wanted a vaginal birth with Lucy, to confirm that my body could work in the normal way, but the midwife said I would have a drip and be monitored throughout labour. She said I would have to sign a disclaimer if I refused and that frightened me. I was too afraid to risk a natural labour in case it went wrong again, so I made the best decision in the circumstances.

'I wasn't ready for a fight so I chose another Caesarean. It was damage limitation, not a positive choice but, looking back, we turned a corner with Lucy's birth. I used osteopathy and homoeopathy to help me recover and realised that I could sort things out for myself. I became more in tune with my body and it felt empowering.

'Perhaps we had to go through Lucy's birth to be able to have

Jack naturally. He was our surprise baby and I was very sick during pregnancy. I couldn't bear the thought of another operation until a friend said, "Why do you need one?"

'I hadn't really thought about it, so I was excited and searched the Internet for information about vaginal birth after a Caesarean. The more I learned, the more confident I felt, and the less I relied on other people.

'I decided not to have the baby in hospital because "trial of labour" sounds so negative. As soon as I made the decision to have a water birth at home my sickness disappeared. Water helps you to relax and gives you privacy, and research suggests that it supports a Caesarean scar by counter-pressure. The preparations became my project for six months.

'I worry about what other people think, so I had to learn to say and do what felt right to me; to trust myself and love my body. I read about and talked to people who had achieved a VBAC. I used homoeopathic remedies and went to cranial osteopathy sessions carrying a lead weight to return not feeling pregnant at all.

'A tense body and a tense mind make for a tight cervix, so I tried to relax and visualise my cervix opening. I talked about "the birth" not "the delivery", which is something that other people do to you. I stuck affirmations around the house so that whenever I opened a cupboard there was a sentence to empower me.

'I requested the notes from my first two labours to help me understand what had happened; and, to avoid spending hours in a crowded waiting room for a five-minute lecture about scar rupture, I sent a polite letter to my consultant.

'The letter said that I intended to have an active home birth and, if he wished, we could arrange a time that was mutually convenient to meet. He didn't reply, but every midwife I met knew about "the letter"!

'I felt I would only let go if everyone could relax and work together, so I tried to think of other people's needs, going for a scan because Jason needed to feel sure that the baby was strong and healthy and getting a prescription for pethidine so that the midwives would know it was there just in case.

'Jason was just as busy at work, but his priorities had changed. We'd gone through some make-or-break situations in the two years before Jack's birth, which gave us the strength and confidence to go ahead. I was afraid of giving birth, but I trusted him and he trusted me, sometimes more than I did myself. Even though it was our third baby, we went to antenatal classes together.

'Everything was our choice, but there were some really low times. At thirty-one weeks, my midwife plunged me into despair by saying that Jack was breech. Jason told me not to panic, we would cross each bridge as we came to it. Jack turned at thirty-four weeks.

'I knew in my heart that I could give birth my way, but I had been belittled by so many doctors in the past that I sometimes doubted myself and needed people to remind me. When you are afraid, your confidence wavers; you need other people to be strong for you. With Jack, I dilated extremely slowly, but it was a mental thing. It hurt so much that I was afraid to let go in case it hurt even more.

'I pushed for over three hours, but I delivered Jack naturally and I finally understood what people mean when they talk about riding the crest of the wave with each contraction. You have to lose control in order to gain control.

'Jason respects me for what we achieved and at first I felt we'd been through something amazing. Now I take it for granted. At times, I felt shaky and unstable in my pelvis, as bad as I had after the Caesareans. You can't put the rest of your life on hold while you bask in the glory of a wonderful birth. A birth is just a part of life.'

Directory

Useful addresses

Association for Improvements in the Maternity Services (AIMS)
5 Ann's Court
Grove Road
Surbiton
Surrey KT6 4BE
UK
Tel: 020 8390 9534
Website: www.aims.org.uk

Birth International
PO Box 366
Camperdown
NSW 1450
Australia
Tel: (02) 9519 5122
Website: birthinternational.com

Health Information Service
UK
Helpline: 0800 665544

Midwifery Today
PO Box 2672-350
Eugene
OR 97402
USA
Website: www.midwiferytoday.com

The National Childbirth Trust (NCT)
Alexandra House
Oldham Terrace
London WC3 6NH
UK
Helpline: 020 8992 8637
Website: www.nct-online.org

Websites

The following provide information for the UK, Australia, Canada, the USA and elsewhere, or links to relevant websites. If you do not find the information you need, contact one of the organisations above.

www.activebirthcentre.com; information on natural and water birth

www.apni.org; for women suffering post-natal illness

www.avma.org; a UK charity offering advice to victims of medical accidents

www.babydirectory.com; local information for pregnant women, babies and children, including pool-hire companies, doulas, independent midwives, hospitals, alternative therapists etc.

www.birthcenters.org; American site with a good selection of links

www.birthchoiceuk.com; up-to-date local information and statistics to help women choose where to give birth in the UK

www.dppi.org; international information service for disabled parents, prospective parents and professionals

www.drfoster.co.uk; an independent organisation providing authoritative information about maternity-service provision

www.homebirth.org; well-respected home-birth reference site which includes research evidence

www.independentmidwives.org; list of UK independent midwives; international contacts

www.internationalmidwives.org; based in the Netherlands, the International Confederation of Midwives site has useful links, including research resources

www.mama.org; groups in the UK to support all mothers, especially those who are lonely or isolated after the birth of a baby or who are moving to a new area

www.midirs.org; information and research evidence for women and midwives

www.midwifery.org; midwives who support women's choices when giving birth

www.patient.co.uk; health information, including Group B strep; click on 'women', then 'pregnancy' or 'childbirth' for links to relevant sites

www.patients-association.com; advice on patient's rights, access to health services, etc

www.sheilakitzinger.com; information about home birth and water birth

www.ukcc.org; maintains professional standards for UK midwives and health visitors. Offers an advice service and deals with complaints

www.vbac.com; American site with advice for women who want to deliver their baby naturally after a Caesarean. Click on 'Support Groups' for UK information

Recommended reading

Enkin, Murray et al, *A Guide to Effective Care in Pregnancy and Childbirth*, third edition, Oxford University Press, 2000. Regularly updated review of the research literature.

Gaskin, Ina May, *Spiritual Midwifery*, The Book Publishing Company, 1990. For inspiration.

Kitzinger, Sheila, *Rediscovering Birth*, Little Brown, 2000. A beautifully illustrated book that asks some searching questions about birth.

National Childbirth Trust, *Caesarean Birth: Your Questions Answered*, National Childbirth Trust, 1996. General information, practical tips and research evidence. Available from NCT – see above.

Thomas, Pat, *Alternative Therapies for Pregnancy and Birth*, Element Books, 2000. Well researched alternatives for women who do not want to be 'patients'.

Thomas, Pat, *Every Woman's Birth Rights*, Thorsons, 1996. Unbiased presentation of facts from the woman's point of view.

Thorn, Gill, *Pregnancy & Birth*, Hamlyn, 2000. General information.

Wesson, Nicky, *Labour Pain*, Vermilion, 1999. Self-help and other methods of pain relief.

Index